T0158176

SAVE
THEM ALL

Allan B Fredrickson

iUniverse, Inc.
Bloomington

SAVE THEM ALL

Copyright © 2011 by Allan B Fredrickson

All rights reserved. No part of this book may be used or reproduced by any means, graphic, electronic, or mechanical, including photocopying, recording, taping or by any information storage retrieval system without the written permission of the publisher except in the case of brief quotations embodied in critical articles and reviews.

The information, ideas, and suggestions in this book are not intended as a substitute for professional medical advice. Before following any suggestions contained in this book, you should consult your personal physician. Neither the author nor the publisher shall be liable or responsible for any loss or damage allegedly arising as a consequence of your use or application of any information or suggestions in this book.

iUniverse books may be ordered through booksellers or by contacting:

iUniverse
1663 Liberty Drive
Bloomington, IN 47403
www.iuniverse.com
1-800-Authors (1-800-288-4677)

Because of the dynamic nature of the Internet, any web addresses or links contained in this book may have changed since publication and may no longer be valid. The views expressed in this work are solely those of the author and do not necessarily reflect the views of the publisher, and the publisher hereby disclaims any responsibility for them.

Any people depicted in stock imagery provided by Thinkstock are models, and such images are being used for illustrative purposes only.

Certain stock imagery © Thinkstock.

ISBN: 978-1-4620-6140-2 (sc)
ISBN: 978-1-4620-6141-9 (e)

Printed in the United States of America

iUniverse rev. date: 12/05/2011

I
dedicate
this book to my daughter
Amy
Not only for her assistance and editing skills
in the writing of this book
but also for her many hours of medical assistance
while working with me at the veterinary
clinic and when making farm calls.

The Cover

The picture on the front cover is an ink drawing done by Yvonne Davis, a Northwest Washington artist, and presented to Dr. Fredrickson as a gift to commemorate the opening of his new veterinary clinic in 1971.

ONE

As he drove south on the old highway, Alton thought how unbelievable it was that Mr. and Mrs. Bill Weber could exist on their small farm that Dr. Friedson estimated to be no bigger than twenty acres, especially when a large part of it contained old buildings, sagging fences, large patches of weeds, and piles of old straw and manure. They were people of the land and they lived on what they could grow and produce. Just west of the house was a small orchard of prune, apple and pear trees and beside it was a large garden bordered on the south side with rhubarb clumps and four long rows of raspberry bushes. The fall months were harvest time; and Mrs. Weber spent many hours over the hot stove canning the fruits and vegetables her efforts produced. Some of the produce was frozen, but most of the space in the large chest freezer was reserved for the meat and poultry produced on the farm and salmon caught in the river that ran past the front of the house.

They had a milking herd of six cows that provided just enough milk to feed the calves and pigs and some milk and cream for the house. They bred each cow every year and each newborn calf was chosen for a purpose. One was raised as a replacement heifer for the oldest cow in the herd, which was then shipped off to the sales market. One was selected to be fattened and butchered for their own use, and the remainder were bred and sold as pregnant heifers to other dairy farmers in the area. The money received from the sales was used for farm expenses and household necessities.

Today Dr. Friedson had an appointment at 10:00 a.m. to check a cow for possible mastitis and castrate a calf that had been chosen to be next year's meat supply.

It was a beautiful sunny spring day and many of the farmers were busy in their fields preparing the rich, black soil for the seeding of peas, spinach, tulip bulbs, potatoes, cabbage cucumbers, and a variety of grains. As he crossed over the narrow steel bridge that spanned the south fork of the Skagit River at the little town of Conway he noticed two boats in the river with four fisherman casting their lines in hope of landing a large Steelhead salmon. At this time of the year the river was quite clean because the winter rains had subsided and the water melting from the mountain snows and glaciers was clear and cold.

As he pulled into the yard, he was met by Curly, an arthritic Chesapeake, who stood wagging his tail and being overly friendly because Dr. Friedson's visit meant he was going to have the opportunity once again to be a referee – to participate in the verbal assault between the goose and the gobbler as they expressed their dissatisfaction of having a stranger trespass through their yard. It was the strangest thing one would have the opportunity to witness. Between the house and the barn was a small patch of grass enclosed by a broken-down, patched-up wooden fence that confined an old gander goose and a hot-tempered turkey gobbler. A dirt path cut through the yard, which was the only way to get from the back of the house to the cattle barn. For some unknown reason that even the Webers couldn't explain, these two usually friendly domestic birds became very upset with each other when someone other than the Webers tried to walk the path to the barn.

The birds would move facing each other on each side of the path and hiss and gobble while poking their beaks at each other in rhythm to the flapping of the wings and stomping of the feet. While this was going on, Curly would back down the path jumping on his hind legs, barking and waving his head, thinking he was the referee and the judge who determined the eventual winner. This circus act would continue until the person passed through the gate at the end of the path. It never failed to happen and was a highlight of making a trip to the Weber farm.

On this particular day, however, the "show stopper" was not the goose and the gobbler act but one that could have been more serious than it was.

When Dr. Friedson entered the barn, Bill Weber greeted him while standing next to Rosie scratching her back and rubbing her neck. It was obvious she was one of his pet cows. He was a short, chubby man and could just barely see over the back of the tall Holstein cow.

"I think she has a touch of mastitis, Doc," Bill said, quick to make a diagnosis. "Her left front quarter had some flakes in the strip cup last night, and this morning the quarter seemed a little hot."

"Did you get any color on the blotter?" Dr. Friedson asked as he knelt by Rosie's right side and slowly ran his hand down her leg and on to her udder.

"No, I didn't have a blotter. I should get a few to have on hand."

Dr. Friedson ran his hand gently around Rosie's udder to detect any abnormalities. She didn't flinch when he squeezed each quarter and there didn't appear to be any difference in size, temperature or firmness between each quarter. He stripped some milk from the left front quarter into his hand, and as he rocked it slowly back and forth he looked closely for any clumps or flakes that would indicate a problem. Seeing none, he reached into his pocket and took out a small piece of blotter paper and squirted a few drops of milk onto each square, then rose to his feet and walked over and stood by Mr. Weber.

"Well, we'll see what the first strip says," Dr. Friedson said holding the blotter up so they both could see it. "I don't see or feel any evidence of mastitis, but if we get color I think we should treat her." Dr. Friedson held the blotter closer to his face and leaned towards the light.

"I think there's a slight change, Bill. I see a little blue." As they stared in anticipation, the upper left square began to change color: first a light blue, then a darker blue and finally a light purple.

"I knew it!" Bill said. "I've been milking these critters for seventy years and I just have a feeling when there is trouble. You better treat her Doc. I'll have to throw the milk but I'll feed it to the pigs."

"Yes, you'll have to hold it for 72 hours," Dr. Friedson replied.

Dr. Friedson went back to his car, hurrying through the yard before the snoozing birds could get their act together, and sorted out the bottles for the treatment. He mixed a dose of antibiotics and drew it into a large syringe and attached a blunt teat needle to the hub. He returned to Rosie, inserted the needle into the teat duct and injected the full amount into the suspect quarter. Rosie shifted her feet as Dr. Friedson vigorously massaged the quarter to distribute the antibiotics into the milk glands and surrounding tissues. As he inserted a plastic teat dilator to plug the duct, he looked at Mr. Weber and said, "Keep that dilator in for 24 hours Bill. I'll leave a couple of test blotters so you can check her progress."

"I know the procedure. Doc Branberg has treated hundreds of these for me over the years. I could do it myself if I had the medicine." He sounded as if his intelligence and capabilities had been insulted.

"Now then, you said you had a bull calf to castrate. Do you have him locked up?"

"Yeah, he's locked in a stanchion in the calf barn."

"Is this one you will fatten and butcher or will you sell him?" Dr. Friedson asked.

"He is the only candidate we have for next year's meat supply. We were lucky this year. We had only one bull calf and four heifers. Millie turned up empty. She must have had an early abortion because I was sure she was pregnant. I have a feeling when they settle. She seems to do this every other year. Maybe I should get rid of her," he talked and waved his hands as they walked towards the calf shed.

"He's tied in here," he said, pointing to an open door.

The procedure Dr. Friedson used to castrate a small calf is the same as that used by most veterinarians across the country. One person positions himself alongside the calf with one leg applying pressure into the calf's flank area. One hand grasps the base of the tail and bends it sharply over the calf's back, serving to semi paralyze the rear legs. The surgeon squats behind the calf, makes a small incision in the bottom of the scrotum and removes the testicles using an emasculator to crush the vessels to reduce excessive bleeding. The procedure is simple, quick and effective. Following the surgery the calf can be released to join his companions in the pasture.

Mr. Weber took his position alongside the calf, and bent its tail sharply over its back. He felt the calf's muscle tense as he pushed in with his knee and put pressure on the tail.

Through tight lips Bill grunted, "Okay, I think I've got him, Doc, go ahead."

Dr. Friedson knelt behind the calf and with scalpel in hand took hold of the scrotum. Just as he made a swipe with the scalpel, Mr. Weber slipped on a piece of wet straw and lost his hold on the tail. Immediately the calf kicked backwards, hitting Dr. Friedson's arms and pushing him sideways. Instead of cutting the bottom of the scrotum, the scalpel sliced across the second joint of Dr. Friedson's left index finger. Dr. Friedson knew the injury was serious. He told Mr. Weber he had cut himself and had to get a bandage, and he hurried to his car. Luckily the taunting birds paid no attention as they lay snoozing in the late morning sun.

After cleaning, treating, and wrapping his hand in sterile gauze, Dr, Friedson leaned against the trunk of his car and slowly went over the events that had just happened knowing he had to make a hasty decision. The bull calf locked in the stanchion still had to be castrated, and Mr., Weber was standing in the barn waiting for the operation to be completed. On the other hand he knew he should get to the hospital and have his hand attended to.

He decided to return to the barn and finish the job at hand so he wouldn't have to return later and fight with a calf that would be several weeks older. By now the goose and gobbler show was ready for him and he had to do some fancy footwork to push through the honking and jabbing and prevent from tripping over the would-be referee.

When he made it back to the barn Mr. Weber was extremely apologetic. "Gosh, I'm sorry Doc. How's the hand? I slipped on a piece of wet straw and lost my hold. Are you going to finish him or should I turn him loose?"

"It's a pretty deep slice but nothing too serious." Dr. Friedson said, hiding his hand so Bill couldn't see the blood seeping through the bandage. "If you can get a hold of him, I would like to finish the job so I don't have to come back later."

In a minute the castration was completed, the calf was turned out to pasture and Dr. Friedson was gathering up his equipment.

"I sure hope you will be okay Doc," Bill said as he stood

leaning against the door. "You better get right to emergency. Being around a barn, those cuts can get infected in a hurry."

"I have one quick stop over on the Bolson Road, then I'll run in and have Dr. Kammon take a look at it," Dr. Friedson said as he picked up his bucket and leather satchel.

As Dr. Kammon applied the last stitch and applied a stabilizing plaster cast, he said, "You know you are pretty lucky. That scalpel blade could have done much more damage to your hand than just that finger. Those blades are extremely sharp. You should be more careful when working around those jittery animals. Keep the cast dry and I want to say don't be too active with that hand but that would be like talking to the wall. Take an aspirin if you need comfort and I'll see you in six weeks."

TWO

The heavy plaster cast on his hand and forearm limited Dr. Friedson's activities that required two good hands, so for the next six weeks most of his time was spent in the hospital tending to small animals in the exam room, doing laboratory procedures, and helping with bookwork. Dr. Branberg was delegated to make all the farm calls and do all the major surgeries. This put him on a tight 24-hour-a- day schedule and he often teasingly said he would eventually get even. He was so busy that most of the elective surgeries such as spays, neuters, tumors, declaws, etc. were postponed until Dr. Friedson was able to use his injured hand.

Rachel was in a state of ecstasy. With Dr. Friedson in the hospital all day, she had someone to jabber to and help with the office work. She had her pet name for both doctors but used them only when clients weren't around. She wanted to be respectful and professional towards the doctors so she didn't use their first names. On the other hand, she considered addressing them with the title of doctor and their surname to be a little stiff and impersonal. As a compromise she settled on Dr. Fried and Dr. B. She even resorted to calling them that when talking to the clients. As will often happen, many of the clients followed her example and began calling Alton by his shortened name - Dr. Fried. It must have been because of his age and professional longevity that none of the clients resorted to the shortened name of Dr. B.

Rachel was in her eighteenth year serving as the receptionist and bookkeeper at the Valley Veterinary Hospital. She was dedicated, efficient, loved her work, and would do anything, short of walking on hot coals, to please the doctors and their clients. Twenty years ago her husband had retired from the navy and, having been stationed at the Whidbey Island Naval Base, they had decided to stay in the area. Her husband had taken a job as a security officer at the Skagit Valley Community College and she had answered the ad for a veterinary receptionist that Dr. Branberg had placed in the Skagit Valley Herald.

When Dr. Branberg interviewed and hired Rachel for the job, he hadn't realized what a gem he was getting. She started slowly but after a few months she turned out to be a hard-working "All-Girl-Friday." Although her job description listed her as the hospital receptionist, she was so ambitious, talented, and efficient she was doing a little bit of everything. She ran the hospital with determination and authority and because she was so successful, the doctors didn't mind stepping back and let her run the ship. She didn't hesitate to correct both doctors if they made a mistake or did something out of line, and they willingly accepted her input because she was courteous, meant well, and always did it in privacy.

One of her many attributes was her ability to recognize and address clients and their pets by their names as soon as they walked in the door. Dr. Friedson, who was notoriously terrible with names, was constantly amazed at how she did it. He took pleasure in telling people how Rachel could meet and talk with a person for only a few minutes, then months later when that person walked into the hospital she would greet them and their pet by their proper name. Many times Dr. Friedson was saved from embarrassment by calling on Rachel's recall talent.

If a long-time client walked in the door and Dr. Friedson couldn't remember their name, he would quickly duck into one of the nearby rooms and quietly motion for Rachel to follow.

"Quickly, tell me, what is her name?" he would whisper.

"That's Mrs. Garley; you should know that!"

"What's the dog's name?"

"Toby; and be careful, he bites," she would warn him.

Dr. Friedson would let Rachel greet the client and visit a little and do the paperwork; then he would walk into the waiting room with a big smile on his face and say confidently, "Well, Mrs. Garley, how are you today? And Toby, what brings you in to see us on this pleasant afternoon?" Mrs. Garley would smile and extend her hand, feeling welcome and pleased with the warm and friendly people at the Valley Veterinary Hospital. Sometimes this scenario repeated itself several times a day with Dr. Friedson often feeling inadequate and embarrassed and Rachel just shaking her head.

THREE

"**G**ood morning, Rachel!" Alton shouted as he walked in the back door. "How's my favorite receptionist today?"

"Don't 'your-favorite-receptionist' me!" she shouted back. "You have a problem and I'm not going to bail you out on this one."

"I can handle it. What's up?"

"Your favorite client, Ben Fraser, called and said he would have his colt Repeater ready for his surgery and he wants you to be on time because he has to be at Longacres by noon," she said with an edge to her voice.

"What's he going to the track for? Did he say?"

"No, but you better call him because you have scheduled a herd pregnancy check out at Smiley's first thing this morning. You know how Ben can be, and if you are not there on time the sparks will fly."

"Well, he was supposed to call me. When I was there checking his mare he said he wanted the colt castrated and he would call to set up an appointment. Did he call earlier?" Alton asked.

"No, he's not on the books, but he's expecting you," she replied.

Alton opened the appointment book and saw that he had the Smiley farm scheduled to pregnancy check some Holstein cows. There was no way he could do that and be at Ben's in time for Ben to be at the track at a decent time. They were both good clients and he didn't want to disappoint either one, so he had to make a decision.

Ben Fraser was extremely difficult to work for because he was demanding, set in his ways, and drew a hard bargain with no room for negotiation. He was a very successful thoroughbred horse breeder and stood one of the best studs in the state, a big bay stud with the registered name of Repeater. He attracted high quality mares and his runners did very well at tracks in and out of the state. Repeater could have been more successful than he was, but Ben was so proud of him he had his breeding fee much too high and was not willing to bargain with owners of exceptional mares. Many times he was so hard to deal with; owners backed down and booked their mares to other studs.

The most frustrating times Dr. Friedson had with Ben was Ben's tendency to want to be the veterinarian and not the client. Every time he called with a problem he had the diagnosis made before Dr. Friedson got there, and he knew exactly how he wanted it handled and treated. This made for some persuasive conversation because he was not always right and what he wanted and suggested was not in the best interest of the horse. Often Dr. Friedson would have to persuade Ben into a more appropriate approach to the problem by telling him outright that he was wrong while being careful not to insult his intelligence. Over the years they learned to respect each other's opinions and developed an amicable relationship. This was a compliment to Dr. Friedson because Ben had chased many veterinarians off his farm, telling them they were incompetent, lacked knowledge, and should have their license revoked.

So it was that Ben expected to have his colt castrated today, and Dr. Friedson better be there to keep Ben a happy client. He dialed the Smiley residence and a male voice answered.

"Hello, Bob, this is Dr. Friedson," he said.

"No, this is Chris," the man interrupted.

"Oh. Hi, Chris. I am calling because I have a scheduling

conflict. I have you down to pregnancy check this morning and I can do it later, but Ben Fraser called and insists I have him down to cut a colt first thing this morning. I would like to do it because you know how Ben can be."

"Hey, everyone knows that what Fraser wants, Fraser gets," Chris replied. "Go ahead, Dr. Fried. I'll wait to put the cows in when you get here. There's no hurry. I have plenty to do."

"Thanks, Chris. I'll see you about ten. Tell your dad I'm sorry about the mix-up."

"Will do," Chris replied and the line went dead.

It was a good time of the year to castrate a stud because it was too early for fly season and late enough that the ground was warm and mostly dry. However, if the cool, cloudy weather brought rain, the surgery would have to be postponed.

Dr. Friedson did all his horse castrations outside on the grass where it was clean, free from dust, with enough room so the horse could get up and stagger around without injuring himself by falling into a wall or fence. The Fraser farm had plenty of clean, short-cut grass to serve as a surgical arena.

Dr. Friedson arrived at the farm in good time and as he pulled into the yard Ben came out of the stud barn carrying a lead rope and a long carriage horse whip. As Dr. Friedson was gathering the scrub pail, soap, disinfectant, scalpel, emasculator, tranquilizer and anesthetic, Ben was explaining to him how to handle the mean farm rooster. "I'll carry your bucket and case and you take this whip. As we walk down the lane, listen for his ruffling because you know how he likes to ruffle his feathers as he runs. When you think he is close enough, turn quickly and crack the whip at him. If you can scare him it may teach him a lesson and make him afraid of you."

Among Ben's flock of Banty chickens was a feisty rooster that liked to attack people when they weren't watching or expecting it. He would lie in wait, and after a person passed him he would attack by pecking and clawing at the person's legs. He had done this to Dr. Friedson several times, tearing his pants and drawing blood. All Dr. Friedson's kicking and hollering hadn't deterred the bird, so Ben thought the whip might be effective.

The two of them walked side by side down the lane and when they were halfway to the shed they heard the swift pitter-patter of feet and the ruffling of feathers as the rooster flapped his wings and ran towards them. Ben took a peek behind and through pursed lips whispered, "Now!" Dr. Friedson whirled, snapped the whip, and then stood motionless with an astonished look on his face as he stared over the fence into the adjacent pasture. When Ben turned around Dr. Friedson put his hands to his head and said, "I think I killed him. Gosh, Ben, I didn't mean to actually hit him. I just wanted to scare him."

When Dr. Friedson turned and flipped the whip, the string on the end wrapped around the rooster's neck and when Dr. Friedson jerked the whip back for another swing, it threw the rooster high into the air, over the fence and into the field. He let out a loud squawk as he landed with a dull thud and then lay motionless. Both men assumed he was dead.

"He's not moving," Ben whispered as he looked over the fence. "Well, he asked for it and he got what he deserved. Don't worry about it. Now I won't have to bother with him. He was a good rooster, though, and I liked having him around."

"I'm sorry. I didn't mean to hurt him," Dr. Friedson said, feeling bad about what had just happened.

With the castration completed and the colt steady on his feet, Dr. Friedson cleaned his equipment and packed it neatly in his car. When he left the farm he turned right onto the Pole Road, heading for the Smiley farm.

Although rectal palpations to determine pregnancies are a

dirty, arm fatiguing-job, it was one of Dr. Friedson's favorite procedures to do on a dairy farm. To be able to confidently announce that a cow was pregnant was not only satisfying to him but it made the farmer happy and made it unnecessary to make a decision about getting rid of the cow if she was empty and a borderline milker.

The scenario was pretty much the same on all the dairy farms in the valley. After several cows in the herd had been bred, either by a bull or by artificial insemination, and had skipped at least two heat cycles, the farmer would call a veterinarian to perform rectal palpations to determine if they had caught and were around 60 days pregnant. On the scheduled appointment day the farmer would put the selected cows in the stanchion shed or milking barn, whichever he used, and the veterinarian would go down the line stating which ones were or were not pregnant. If the veterinarian was experienced and had a good touch, the exam was almost 100% effective, and if the cow was pronounced pregnant at the time but came up empty after nine months, it was usually because she aborted, not because the doctor made a mistake.

After many months of practice on hundreds of cows, a veterinarian could insert his arm into the rectum of a cow, pick up and palpate her uterus and make a decision in less than a minute. If the cow cooperated by relaxing and standing still, the procedure was quick, simple and effective. The veterinarian would put on a shoulder-length rubber or plastic sleeve on his arm, lubricate it with a gel, and insert his arm up the cow's rectum, pushing aside the bladder and intestines to locate the uterus and ovaries. Most times he had to scoop out several handfuls of feces to make room for his arm. Then locating the ovary, he would cup his hand around the uterus and follow it down towards the body of the uterus near the cervix. This was repeated on both the left and right horns of the uterus. If the cow was around 60 days pregnant he would feel a firm, round swelling about the size of a grapefruit in one of the horns. If one could see it, it would look like a snake that had just swallowed a rat. Following a successful palpation he would declare her pregnant or barren, withdraw his arm and go on to the next cow. This would continue until all the cows had been palpated.

The farmer would make a notation on a calendar when she was due and when she should be taken out of the milking string in preparation for the calving. If all went normally, she would freshen in seven months, delivering a strong, healthy calf, and return to the milking string to repeat the procedure all over again. The dairy farmer's business and livelihood was almost 100% dependent on his cows getting pregnant year after year.

FOUR

I t was a beautiful sunny morning and Alton was on his way back to the hospital after Bangs testing a herd of cattle for tuberculosis when Rachel's voice broke on the radio, "This is 963 calling 201, 963 calling 201, over."

"This is 201. How is Rachel this morning?" Alton answered cheerfully.

"I'm my usual pleasant self," she said, trying to be upbeat. "On your way in you better stop at Ben Fraser's. He said the colt you castrated is all humped up and has a bad case of colic. He says he needs you right away."

"If he's standing around all humped up, it isn't colic. He's not draining. Did Ben say anything about the incision?"

"He didn't say. You know Ben. He made the diagnosis and wants you to treat the colt for colic."

"Well, this is going to be fun," Alton said sarcastically. "I'll have to use my strongest persuasive powers to convince him I'll have to open the incision, and he'll still want me to treat the colt for colic. I'll swing over there. I'm just coming up to the Highway 9 Bridge. Call and tell him I'll be there in fifteen minutes. 201 is out."

The most important aftercare on a colt castration is keeping the incision open for at least three days to allow the tissues to drain the fluid that tends to collect resulting from the trauma caused by the procedure. If the edges of the skin at the bottom of the scrotum heal together too quickly, edematous fluid collects, causing swelling, pain and possible infection. This can be prevented by vigorously exercising the colt twice a day by walking or gypping which prevents the incision from closing too soon. Ben Fraser had had dozens of colts castrated and knew the procedure as well as anyone in the horse business. He would be deeply offended if told, or even if it was implied, that the problem was not intestinal colic but pain due to scrotal swelling because of neglect or improper aftercare. Alton was wondering how he could tactfully suggest opening the incision while pretending to treat the colt for colic.

Upon a quick examination Dr. Friedson could find no concrete evidence that the yearling was experiencing pain due to intestinal colic. There had been no rolling in the stall, stomping of the feet, extension of the head and neck, and no extended firmness in the abdomen. When auscultating the intestines he heard normal sounds of movement and contractions and no audible sounds of grunting or heavy breathing. The horse was not exhibiting a typical bout of colic.

Although Dr. Friedson was going through the procedure of examining for colic, he was also paying attention to the colt's posture and sneaking a peek at the scrotum for evidence that the castration incision was draining properly. It didn't take long for him to conclude that the problem was not a case of colic but a buildup of fluid in the inguinal area, causing the colt to stand stiff legged, reluctant to move and not eat his daily ration. Dr. Friedson would have to open the incision but the question weighing heavily on his mind was how he was going to convince Ben that he was wrong on his diagnosis and hadn't exercised the colt adequately. Although he already knew the consequences, Dr. Friedson decided to be upfront and tell Ben directly and back up his diagnosis with the visible evidence. If Ben chose to be difficult and not believe him, then so be it.

He looked Ben directly in the eye and said, "This is not a case of colic, Ben, he's stove up from the pressure in the scrotum. I'll open it…."

"Don't you touch that incision!" Ben interrupted with a bit of anger in his voice. "There's nothing wrong with the castration. He has colic and will be fine after treatment and some walking. I know colic when I see it."

"I tend to disagree. Look, Ben, there is no rolling, his nostrils aren't flared, there's intestinal gurgling and there's a fresh pile of manure in the corner of the coral. I'll spread the incision, you walk him a little and he'll be fine."

"Are you going to do it my way or not?" Ben insisted.

Dr. Friedson stood his ground. "Giving him a relaxant and oil won't do any good. In fact it will make the situation worse. If he's not opened up he could get an infection and then he'll really be in trouble."

"Then pack up your things and leave. I'll get someone who knows what they're doing," he said as he walked towards the gate.

"Listen, Ben," Dr. Friedson tried to reason. "Okay, it's your horse. I'll treat him for colic as you say, but I also have to flush out that incision."

"Get in your car and leave. I don't have time. I have to make some phone calls," he turned and walked swiftly to the house. As he reached the door he hollered back and said, "By the way, you didn't kill that rooster. I saw him later that day up walking around. He was a little dizzy. He didn't show up today so I think you taught him a lesson."

Although the rooster's condition was good news, Dr. Friedson stood dejectedly in the open barnyard hoping Ben would change his mind, but he just kept walking and slammed the door as he entered the house.

FIVE

D r. Friedson climbed into his car and slowly drove back to the hospital. He felt badly about what had happened but he was proud of himself for not giving in by doing something he knew was not right. The colt did not have intestinal colic so he couldn't die from such a condition, exposing Dr. Friedson to a charge of neglect. If the colt suffered severe complications from lack of care following the castration, Ben could not come back to Dr. Friedson and reprimand him for not handling the case properly and doing what needed to be done. He hoped that as the day went by, Ben Fraser would recognize his mistake, get someone to properly treat the colt, and maybe be man enough to call Dr. Friedson and apologize for his behavior. He knew this was wishful thinking.

When Alton walked in the back door of the hospital, Dr. Branberg had his car keys in his hand and was putting on his hat to leave. "I guess I have to take care of Ben Fraser's horse. He called and said the colt had colic and you refused to treat him. You insisted that his condition had nothing to do with colic and that you wanted to open the castration incision."

"That Ben can sure be a hardhead," Alton said, slamming his billing case on the desk. "That colt's belly is as normal as mine and he wants me to pump him full of colic medicine. It won't the colt any good and tomorrow he will be so stoved up he won't be able to walk. Ben won't let me touch the incision. Maybe you will have better luck with him."

"He wasn't in a very pleasant mood when he called," Rachel added. "My guess is that he will not have you out again."

"Just wait until he has an emergency on a difficult case and he can't get anyone to look at it or know how to treat it, he'll come calling and be as sweet as sugar," Dr. Friedson said sarcastically.

"Will you go if that happens?" Rachel asked.

"Of course. I took the veterinarian's oath and it is my duty to care for the animals no matter what kind of a jackass the owner turns out to be."

As Dr. Branberg reached for the door knob, he let out a deep sigh and said, "Well, I'll get the incision open and draining even if I have to go over Ben's head."

"You better give him some antibiotics; it's been almost four days," Alton called after him.

The events of the visit to the farm were predictable. As the men walked to the corral, Mr. Fraser would tell Dr. Branberg what an incompetent associate he had in Dr. Friedson and he should think about replacing him and getting a good horse doctor. Dr. Branberg would shrug and hold his tongue. After his examination Dr. Branberg would agree that the colt had some minor signs of colic and should have a little treatment, upon which he would give minimum dosages except for a large dose of antibiotics. As a routine procedure he would suggest checking the scrotum and while he had his hand in position he would quickly open the incision allowing the wound to drain. He would say, as if to himself, that the procedure needed to be done and that the swelling should be down in a couple of days. He would give instructions for Ben to walk the colt three times a day until the symptoms dissipated.

Only time would tell if Dr. Friedson would ever again set foot on the Fraser Thoroughbred Farm.

SIX

Alton didn't grow up on a farm, but had several uncles who farmed within a few miles of each other and he and his siblings visited and worked on the farms whenever feasible. He had one brother and four sisters, and they couldn't wait for school to be out so they could head to the farms for the summer. One of the uncles would pick the family up and take them to one of the farms where they would stay for most of the summer. Alton usually worked for his uncle Orlin who had a big farm and needed additional help caring for the animals, putting up hay, working the summer fallow, and helping with the grain harvest.

Alton loved all aspects of farming but really enjoyed working with and around the animals. Driving the tractor was fun but if he had a preference he would hitch up the horses and rake hay, haul bales or pick stones from the fields. His favorite chore was to saddle up one of the riding horses and ride over to the summer pasture to check on the beef cows and fill the watering tank. He would pretend to be a cowboy herding the cattle down the Chisholm Trail, fighting off rustlers, and rounding up the strays.

Uncle Orlin had just about every domestic bird and animal a small farm could handle. There were horses and colts, cows and calves, pigs, a few sheep, lots of chickens and ducks and even a few turkeys. They all needed to be fed and cared for, and as Alton got older he took it upon himself to be their caretaker. Uncle Orlin was experienced in animal husbandry and patiently taught Alton useful skills and showed him what to look for to keep the animals healthy and productive. Thus was laid the groundwork for Alton's profession as a veterinarian.

The first year out of high school, Alton worked on his uncle Orlin's farm during the summer then enrolled in the engineering curriculum at the local Community College. At the beginning of his second year he was drafted into the United States army and served several months in Korea towards the tail end of the war. He didn't especially like the army, but upon his discharge he qualified for the GI Bill enabling him to continue his education. He graduated with a BS degree in animal husbandry from the University of Minnesota with a specialization in artificial breeding. However, to his disappointment, this was a relatively new field in the animal business and none of the inseminating companies were hiring. He had a valuable diploma but couldn't get a job in his studies.

As fate would have it, everything was to work out to his benefit. During his senior year he lived in a fraternity house with several friends who were studying to be veterinarians. They constantly encouraged Alton to apply to the College of Veterinary Medicine and study to get his doctorate. His reply was always the same, "I am not smart enough and would never make it."

After much praying, talking to his parents and consulting with his school counselors, he decided to submit his application to the College of Veterinary Medicine. He then went to work for his uncle Clary in North Dakota while waiting for a reply. His uncle Clary had just had drastic stomach surgery and needed help running his farm. It was late in the summer and Alton was on the tractor baling straw when he saw his cousin running across the field waving what was obviously a letter. When he stopped the tractor Jerome showed him the envelope and said, "It's from the college; the Veterinary College! They're letting you know you can go to school there and become a doctor."

Alton stared at the envelope for the longest time.

"Open it, open it!" Jerome yelled as he jumped on the wheel of the tractor.

Alton's heart began to beat a hundred miles an hour, beads of sweat formed on his brow and his hands began to shake. At that moment he knew that he wanted to be a veterinarian more than anything in the world. Up until now he thought he could take it or leave it but now, with the decision in his hand, he knew he would be devastated if rejected. Slowly he tore the end of the envelope open and blew in the end to separate the edges. He looked in and saw a single piece of paper folded into thirds. He pulled it out, opened the top flap and the first word he saw was Congratulations! He froze. He couldn't move, he couldn't speak. He was oblivious to Jerome tugging at his arm asking, "What does it say, what does it say?"

The letter went on to say he had been accepted into the College of Veterinary Medicine and would be welcomed into the fall class beginning 8:00 a.m. September 16.

The first year was a struggle, but he made it through although he was rated in the lower one tenth of the class. His second year began with trouble brewing on the horizon and when he returned after Christmas for the second quarter of class, he was informed that he was being flunked out of the class because his grades were inadequate. Although it was a shock, he wasn't surprised considering the circumstances. He made a promise to himself that he would be back.

During the previous summer he had found out that his mother was diagnosed with an advanced case of uterine cancer which had spread to other abdominal organs. She was given less than a year to live. He left for school in September knowing he may have seen his mother for the last time. His GI Bill had run out and he didn't make nearly enough money during the summer to see him through a year of school. To meet his expenses he worked two night jobs involving four nights a week and a Saturday job. This left very little time for study. He couldn't afford to buy text books, which meant he had to use the library but it closed at 10:00 p.m. when he was just getting off work. With the worry and concern about his mother, his financial woes and lack of study time, he could not keep his grades up and stay up with his class, so he had to drop out for the year.

As it turned out, it was the best thing that could have happened to him. He was able to get a good, well paying job, he and his fiancé were married the following summer, he was reinstated into the Veterinary College, and with his wife working and him having a part-time job at the school, there were no distractions and he was able to concentrate on his studies. In three years he graduated with his DVM and even though he was rated in the lower end of his class, he was proud of his accomplishment.

Within six weeks, his family, including their two year-old son, was settled in their new home and Alton was hired into what he considered the ideal practice with a once-in-a-life-time associate.

SEVEN

Mount Vernon is a small but bustling town that straddles the Skagit River just before the icy waters flow into Skagit Bay. The town is the shopping hub of the county and the downtown streets are usually full of cars and shoppers late into the evening. The river flows through the valleys and gullies along the western slopes of the Cascade Mountains then spreads out as it meanders through several miles of flat lands and through the heart of Mount Vernon before emptying into the bay.

Before dozens of engineers and contractors built the levees and dikes, the river often flooded the floor of the Skagit valley with several feet of water, depositing sand and silt as it receded; leaving the farmland soils some of the richest and most fertile in the country. Farmers plant and harvest a wide variety of grains, fruits, vegetables, flower bulbs, and vegetable seeds. The dairymen have lush pastures for their Holsteins, Guernseys, and Jerseys, and the ranchers have adequate grass and hay for their livestock.

Because of its diversified resources, Skagit County is widely known for its stable economy and opportunity for employment. People travel from around the world to work in the forests and lumber mills, the fish hatcheries and canneries, the farms and ranches, recreation endeavors, and the retail trades. The area has a lot to offer both for commerce and recreation, and people take advantage of it.

Mount Vernon is a growing community: each New Year

sees an increase in population, new houses, and several startup businesses. The residents, both old and new, excitedly welcome any and all new businesses and give them their full support and encouragement. When someone hears that a new clothing store or national restaurant chain is coming to town, the word spreads rapidly and the local newspaper makes the announcement with a front page article. When the paper published an article that Doctor Blayne was going to open a veterinary clinic on the south edge of town, Dr. Branberg and Dr. Friedson welcomed the news even though they knew it would be in competition with their own practice.

The town has just about everything a community could want or need for shopping, services, medical needs, recreational, and cultural activities. It isn't necessary for people to travel the sixty or seventy miles to one of the bigger cities to shop, although some do when shopping for a high priced item such as a car, thinking they may have a larger selection and get a better deal.

The downtown area of Mount Vernon consists of four, five-block-long streets running parallel to the river. The buildings are crowded together and the owners announce and advertise their businesses with bold signs hanging over the sidewalks and with bright letters and pictures painted on the windows. There are no dilapidated or boarded up stores, and the city prunes and cares for the many deciduous trees planted along the sidewalks to beautify and offer shade to the downtown area. There are restaurants, clothing shops, lawyers, realtors, banks, and beauty salons on every street and many smaller businesses on the side streets. The town has two hardware stores, a Sears and Penney's department store, three furniture stores and three theaters. Safeway is the largest grocery store but there are several Mom and Pop markets on corners around town. On the outskirts of the town proper are three lumber yards, five gas stations, five auto dealerships along with several used-car lots.

The town boasts of having a modern, up-to-date hospital surrounded by many professional medical and dental clinics staffed with excellent doctors and nurses. Carnation operates a milk condensary on the north end along the river, and Dairygold has a milk bottling and butter making plant on the south end. These comprise the two largest industries in the community. The Chamber of Commerce is quick to note that Mount Vernon has an airport capable of handling small aircraft.

The town of 12,000 people has four elementary schools, one junior high school, and one high school that graduates an average of 200 students each spring. On the northeast corner of town sits the Skagit Valley Community College campus with an enrollment of 1600 full-time students and the facilities to entertain the community with plays, concerts, and other cultural programs. There are 33 churches scattered around the community with the most conspicuous being the First Baptist Church that sits on the hill just above the railroad tracks and rings the time of day every hour with the large bells hanging in the church tower.

The community would not be complete without the busy drinking establishments, and it's hard to miss the bars and lounges with their bright neon lights and sidewalk sandwich boards advertising their products. Scotty's Pool Hall with its thirteen green felt tables borders the south end of Third Street, and Cedar Dance Hall is considered the north end of Fourth Street. Dances are held every Friday and Saturday night and the place is usually packed. The young lumberjacks and wealthy fishermen are ready for a weekend of fun and The Cedars provides the playground.

The predominant residential housing lies to the east of the business district and is slowly creeping up the slopes of the Cascade foothills as new houses are being built. The street numbers get higher as one travels east and the city limits have been extended to 20th Street which, to most residents, seems to be a long way out of town.

The Valley Veterinary Hospital is situated on the west side of the Skagit River, fronting the main road leading out of town. Because the lowland is subject to flooding, this smaller developed area consists of only a few businesses and some small, older homes. At one time it was a busy retail hub of the community, but because of the slow and congested one-way traffic across the narrow bridge, people are reluctant to set up business there, preferring the heavier traffic volume along the interstate highway running through the downtown area.

The residents of Mount Vernon are proud of their community and willingly participate in the many local programs, projects, and activities to strengthen and perpetuate the friendly progressive feeling that exists throughout the town. The "old-timers" vehemenently argue that because of its beautiful setting, the friendly down-to-earth people, the comfortable year-round weather, and the economic and recreational opportunities, Mount Vernon is "Heaven on Earth."

EIGHT

"I'll give him the message and if he is still here at 5:00 I'll kick him out the door." Rachel hung up the phone and walked directly into the surgery.

"Bev called to remind you that Allan has a baseball game at 5:30 today and he is pitching so it would be nice if you would be there. She is going to drop him off at the PUD Park, then take Ann and Marie to Alice's piano lesson. She will meet you at the game after the lesson." Her voice got weaker as she watched blood oozing from the eye of a Pekinese Dr. Friedson was working on.

"I'll be there. He's a pretty good pitcher and I enjoy watching him play."

Alton and Bev had just celebrated their tenth wedding anniversary and lived in a big frame house on a ninety-acre farm two miles north of town in the Nookachamps Creek area. When they decided to buy a place they hadn't been looking for that much acreage but it was a good location and the price was affordable. The owners, Mr. and Mrs. Wallup, wanted to sell and move in a hurry, so they reduced the price and gave the Friedsons a deal they couldn't refuse. Mr. Wallup was suffering from Parkinson's disease and his doctor told him if he didn't get away from the stress and maintenance of the farm he would probably die in a few years. Mrs. Wallup put her foot down and said, "We are leaving this place even if we have to give it away." The two parties sat down and in less than an hour had agreed to a rough contract. The agreed-upon price for the land and buildings was $46,000, with the Wallups carrying two contracts in order for the agreement to be workable for the Friedsons. They would begin paying on the first $23,000 at an interest rate of 3% with the second $23,000 bearing no interest until the first contract was fully paid. This made the Friedson's payments affordable, and the Wallups were able to quickly sell the farm and move to a smaller home in town and have a monthly income for many years. The papers were signed and the Friedsons with their two children, Allan age 6 and Alice 3, moved into their new home. Bev had just become pregnant with their third child, due to deliver the following spring. Marie was born in April and three years later Ann was born in May.

Purchasing the Wallup farm turned out to be a wise and wonderful purchase for the family. It provided room for the kids to romp and play and to have a large variety of animals to occupy their time and teach them responsibilities. There were many dogs and cats, chickens, pigs, goats, cows, and except for Bev, each family member had a horse to ride and care for. Alton had a couple of thoroughbred broodmares, which he bred to local studs and sold the yearlings at the fall Thoroughbred Select sale. He never produced an outstanding runner but it was a fun hobby for him and did provide some extra income.

Some of the land was rented to neighboring farmers to grow grass and corn to feed their cows and other livestock. At different times three parcels of land were sold to friends to build a house and have a few acres for a garden and a dog or two. Allan had a Red Shorthorn cow in a 4-H program and had a good experience showing her at the local fair. She proved to be a little unruly but he managed to keep her under control and was proud to take home a placing ribbon.

The only disadvantage of living out of town was all the driving Bev had to do as all four children took music lessons, were heavily involved in school, sports and community activities; and of course wanted to spend more time with their friends. She did most of the "taxi" driving as Alton was tied up working long days and many weekends. Many times he had to miss a baseball game or band concert or leave a soccer game, basketball tournament or school play to attend to an emergency.

Alton loved the farm and because of it his family and friends termed him a workaholic. The acreage, buildings, fences, and animals gave him the opportunity to get away from the stress and rigors of a busy medical practice and get down and dirty while farming, which was dear to his heart. There was so much to do and little time to do it. Not that some things had to get done and there was a timetable, but he took pride in the farm and became restless when a project was unfinished, something was broken or out of place, or a new project was waiting to get started. Because of his farm experiences as a young boy, he was pretty much a jack-of-all-trades and was capable of building and repairing most anything connected with the farm and its operation.

He solicited help from friends when necessary and hired someone for a job only if he didn't have the tools or equipment to do it. He had to hire a contractor when it was necessary to put in a new road to the house and paid a well drilling company to install an immersable pump into the well. Otherwise he did everything himself. With building and repairing sheds and barns, putting up fences, doing field work, planting shrubs and flowers, mowing grass, and caring for the animals it would be easy for him to be a full-time farmer, but, as it was meant to be, he had another more important occupation.

NINE

Alton had told Bev many times that the most pleasant part of every day was slipping into bed and cuddling next to her soft, warm, curled up body, then lying quietly sensing the rhythmic rise and fall of her chest with each restful breath. Most nights he retired before her (she tended to be a night owl) and fell asleep before she got into bed so he didn't always get to experience the comfort and togetherness that he found so relaxing. But when he had a late call and she was in bed when he got home, he tenderly wrapped his arms around her and got in a few minutes of snuggling before falling quickly to sleep.

Sometimes Bev would be awake when he crawled into bed, and they would take the opportunity to share their day's activities and she would often remind him of the family events happening the next day that he should be aware of.

Alton was constantly impressed with how Bev managed the four children, prepared the meals, kept the house in order, shuttled the kids around to their activities and still made time for her friends and her interests. She was an accomplished musician and was often asked to accompany soloists and instrumentalists, entertain at parties and gatherings, and play at weddings and funerals. She was the accompanist for one of the local chorales, which consisted of over one hundred singers and she was the choir director and substitute organist at the First Presbyterian Church. The amazing thing about all of it was she did it on a tight budget and on an average of six hours of sleep a night. He often wondered how she did it.

Most of their talks and discussions centered on the family. Seldom did they discuss Alton's work, and if they did it was in generalities and nothing very specific. There was the odd time when he would relate a funny incident or an extremely odd case that he thought Bev might be interested in, or he would tell her about an unusual event if he seemed upset and she asked about it. Otherwise he didn't bring his work home and Dr. Branberg preferred that the wives didn't get involved in the hospital and in the happenings of the practice. When clients called Alton at home and Bev answered the phone, she seldom entered into a conversation about the nature of the call and carried on a conversation only if she knew the client personally.

There were a few occasions, however, when Alton requested her involvement. There was a client, George Ralston, who always trailered his horses to the Friedson farm when he had a problem. He commuted 64 miles one way to work so was never home during the day, so if a horse needed veterinary care it had to be in the evening. He tried to be accommodating by bringing the horse to Alton's farm so he wouldn't have to drive all the way out to his place after work. The problem was George liked to talk, and after the horse's problem was taken care of he wanted to sit on the tailgate and discuss all the issues of the world. Alton wanted him to get in his truck and go home. He had already put in a full day, and not that George's stories were boring and uninteresting, but he tended to tell the same ones over and over again. Alton knew he was in for a long session when George would ease himself down onto the fender of the trailer with a long sigh and reach into his shirt pocket for a hand-rolled cigarette. The first words out of his mouth were, "Well, you know, Doc," he would say with his slow drawl as he lit the smoke, pushed his hat back on his head and leaned back ready to give his views on any subject that came to mind.

Alton and Bev had devised a plan to prevent Alton from getting into this time-wasting predicament when Alton had a schedule to keep and didn't want to be abrupt or rude in telling George he didn't have time to visit. Bev would watch out the kitchen window, and when she saw George sit down on the fender of the trailer and reach for a cigarette, she would step out the back door and shout, "Alton, I need you in here, now!" Alton would excuse himself by saying he should probably get in the house and help with the kids; he would say goodbye to George and slowly walk away. George would get a disappointed look on his face, climb into his truck and slowly turn the vehicle around, watching and hoping Doc would come back out before he got away.

TEN

As Alton Friedson drove his 1965 blue Ford car out of the barnyard he had a puffed-up feeling of satisfaction. He thought how fortunate he was to have the education, the opportunity and the desire to ease the suffering and save the lives of both domestic and wild creatures. It is something that few people get to experience. Long before he was a veterinarian, practically as long as he could remember, he had spent as much time as possible working with and caring for animals, getting close to the dogs and cats of his friends and neighbors and all the animals on his uncles' farms. During his school years he had spent every summer on one of the farms owned by his mother's brothers, and although most of his responsibilities were doing chores around the house and barns, his favorite activities were centered around the animals. He gave every farm animal and bird a name and he knew every one of them by its characteristics or its actions and attitude.

Alton loved to feed the calves and would rap them on the nose when they turned to suck their buddy's ears after downing a bucket of milk. He kicked at the pigs when they tried to hog the feed trough and pushed others away from the milk and grain mash. He rolled in the grass and played with the piglets while their mothers expressed their concerns with grunts and squeals while being barricaded behind the pigpen boards.

One of his daily chores was to feed the chickens and gather the eggs. When he called them in with his familiar whistle, the chickens came running to peck at the corn and ground grains with their mothers hurrying them along so as not to miss the better part of the meal. While they were distracted with their eating, Alton would search for the eggs. He knew where all the nests were hidden and how many eggs there should be, provided each hen laid an egg a day.

Over the years Alton learned that a hen does not always lay an egg every day. Most of them will skip a day once a week. He knew that with twenty laying hens he was going to get, on average, sixteen eggs a day. Some days he gathered nineteen or twenty and on other days he may get only fourteen. If several hens decided to set their eggs, then the count went down considerably. The eggs that weren't used in the house for cooking and baking were taken to town on Saturday, along with the sweet cream, and sold for grocery money. Aunt Louella was always happy when the hens had a good week.

His most fun part of the day was when he had time to spend time with the horses. His uncle Olin had three workhorses and two riding horses and when they weren't being worked, and when Alton had finished his chores, he was permitted to go riding. Chief was a big-boned bay gelding, with head and feet that seemed too big for his short, slim body. He had a lazy streak and was not a happy horse when taken from his afternoon nap to go galloping through the fields. Alton's favorite was a little black mare called Bella. After picking her feet, brushing her shiny black coat, combing her long mane and tail, and strapping on a straight bit bridle, he would ride for hours through the hay meadows. Alton chased his fantasies and Bella seemed more than happy to go along with the games until exhaustion caught up with them both and they'd have to stop to catch their breath. They could easily waste away an afternoon running with the wind and the birds, enjoying each other's company until time to herd in the cows for the evening milking.

As much as Alton thought of the farm as a petting zoo and an amusement park, he was aware of the reality of life and accepted the disappointments and heartaches that went along with being associated with animals. In his younger years it was difficult for him, but he understood that many of the livestock were raised for food and would eventually be butchered to feed the family. He often cried when a chicken was killed for a Sunday dinner or a pet pig or pet calf was slaughtered and put in the locker. It didn't bother him too much when a steer was selected because the beef cattle grazed in the summer pasture away from the barnyard and he seldom came in contact with them. But he often had nightmares when it was a pig or lamb that was chosen and he was around to hear the shot and witness the cutting. When Uncle Olin told him that Snorkel or Sloppy or Bandy was to be put down the next day, he would have a restless night

It was especially hard on him when Snoot was chosen to become the hams, chops, and bacon for the following winter's dinners. Snoot was born the runty pig of a large litter and was too little and weak to fight for a nipple and had to be fed with a bottle until he was big enough to hold his own. Alton took on the job of feeding and caring for the little outcast, which meant fixing a bottle of milk several times a day and patiently holding it until the piglet had his belly full. It was impossible not to get attached to the tiny pig, and as time went by, the two of them bonded like brothers. But, as time has proven, all things must come to an end, and as Snoot developed into a feeder pig and then into a fat butcher hog, his time was limited and his fate predictable. If he had been born a female he may have been chosen as a replacement brood sow, but being a castrated male, he was destined for the meat locker.

On the morning Snoot was to be taken from his friends, Alton took him to a quiet spot in the woods behind the duck pond to play together and have time to say goodbye. As he scratched the pig's belly and rubbed his ears, Snoot looked up at him and grunted as if he understood every word that was being said. Alton explained to him that pigs were born to be fattened and butchered to provide food for people so they could do what people do. It was the same for the cows, the sheep, the chickens and turkeys. They would be sacrificed so others could live.

When it was time to go, Alton wrapped his arms around Snoot's short, bristly neck, and with tears in his eyes, said goodbye one last time and led him back to the yard and slowly shut the door to the holding pen. It broke his heart, and he knew he would sneak off several times during the next week and cry silently to himself. During these lonely, sobbing, heart-wrenching times he would ask over and over again, "Why did it have to be?"

ELEVEN

Of all the modern day appliances in the home, the equipment in the office and the handy gadgets for convenient living, Alton considered the telephone to be the most irritating and the one he would most like to get rid of, if he had a choice. The machine seemed to be the major cause for disruption and edginess in his life 24/7.

He jumped every time the phone rang. And even though only a few calls were for business purposes, he assumed every ring signaled an emergency. Many times he had to leave the family, quit a project, postpone an outing, or, worst of all, crawl out of a nice, warm bed where he'd snuggled next to his wife, to attend to his clients' needs. He swore that if he kept a ledger, he could prove that most emergencies came at the most inconvenient times. Many times, while watching TV, he had to miss the last part of an exciting football game, the climax of a mystery program, or the last episode of an interesting serial. He missed many of the children's activities, parties, and his personal appointments, all because of his dedication and commitment to his practice. When on call at nights and weekends, he often felt guilty when leaving the house because of the possibility a client may have an emergency and the office would not be able to reach him. It was his responsibility to be available while he was on call, and yet he had responsibilities to his family and private life that needed attention. This meant it was not reasonable to just stay at home thinking the phone might ring.

He disliked the phone so much he rarely answered it when it

rang. He could be sitting right next to it and wouldn't pick it up unless he was sure no member of the family was available to do so.

Alton found it interesting when talking to some of his professional friends that most of them had a similar aversion to the telephone. Although they admitted that the monster was essential for a successful business, they would be more at ease if it weren't in their homes. An orthodontist friend said he lived in fear that an emergency call would come just when it was important for him to attend to something involving the family.

A veterinary colleague told Alton about an emergency that came in when his wife was in labor with their first child. She was having contractions and they were getting ready to leave the house when the phone rang. He didn't want to answer it but he was on call and was obligated. It turned out that a dog had been hit on the highway and a county sheriff had picked it up and was on his way to the doctor's clinic. The sheriff radioed his office with instructions for the dispatcher to call the veterinarian to meet him there. The doctor told the dispatcher she would have to try to get someone else because he was taking his wife to the hospital and didn't have time to help. The sheriff waited at the hospital but no doctor was immediately available, and the dog died.

Unbeknownst to the veterinarian, the dog belonged to one of the clinic's best dairy clients. He was terribly upset over the incident and never did business with the clinic after that. The veterinarian was extremely apologetic, but the client put his farm dog above the doctor's family and wouldn't listen to reason Alton told his friend that if that was the kind of person the client was, he shouldn't agonize over losing him and the business was better off without him.

One of the worst fears a doctor lives with while practicing medicine is to be proven negligent. There are few things more damaging in a lawsuit than to be found willfully negligent while attending to a case. If a doctor performs to the best of his knowledge and ability, that is all that can be asked of him. But if a client can prove that the doctor didn't do what he was capable of and neglected to do what he knew was right, then he could be in trouble. Many people in the medical profession have paid dearly and even lost their licenses because they were negligent.

Dr. Friedson was in that position once and it scared him so much he swore it would never happen again.

TWELVE

It was Sunday morning and the family was hurrying to finish breakfast and get ready for church.

"Alton, I laid Ann's clothes out on the bed. That shirt buttons down the back, not the front. I know she doesn't like those white shoes but convince her to wear them. Those black ones are all scuffed," Bev called from the bathroom as she ran the water for her bath.

It was a special Sunday at the Presbyterian Church because it was Youth Sunday and the children were going to participate in the service. The three older children were involved and had been rehearsing for several weeks in Sunday school and at home.

Allan was to be the father in a short skit about the Prodigal Son and had a solo in the children's choir anthem. Alice had been chosen to lead the congregation in the call to confession and was to be one of the Egyptian peasants in the skit. Marie was excited but also nervous because she was to be a candle lighter for the candles on the back of the chancel screen and she was afraid she might stumble and set the church on fire. At night she would lie in bed and say, "But Dad, what if I stumble going up the steps? You know how clumsy I am."

The family belonged to The First Presbyterian Church, located on a full block across from the hospital on the east side of town. The children loved their Sunday school classes and would run down the hall to their rooms to greet their friends and tell the teacher of any interesting event that may have happened during the week. After an hour in their classes the children joined their parents for the morning worship service. Or went to child care if the parents so chose.

Alton and Bev were very active in the church, and a large part of their social activities revolved around church programs and activities. Alton sang bass in the choir, was a substitute Sunday school teacher and served on the Building and Grounds Committee. He used his handyman skills to replace, repair, rebuild or repaint anything that needed attention inside or outside the building. Although he grew up a Lutheran, he was happy and comfortable with the Presbyterian liturgy and theology.

In the church, Bev found an outlet for her musical skills and knowledge. She served on the Worship and Music Committee, was the substitute organist and the assistant choir director. On Sundays when she wasn't playing or directing, she sang alto in the choir. She loved to assist in choosing the hymns and anthems for the Sunday services and would practice them on the piano at home. An excellent musician, playing the piano or organ, at church or home, was fulfilling for her.

As usual it took some time and a group effort to get everyone ready to head out the door, into the Ford station wagon and on to the church. The children were dressed in their Sunday outfits, Bev was putting the finishing touch on her makeup, and Alton had just settled into his easy chair with the sports page of the morning paper when the telephone rang. As she always did, Alice rushed to answer it, thinking it would be one of her friends. In her mind she was the most popular member of the family and most of the calls were for her. When she didn't begin jabbering right away, Alton knew it was for him – the dreaded emergency.

"It's for you, Dad," she said, laying the phone on the desk.

"Hello," he said, trying to be cheerful even though he knew what the caller was going to say.

"Dr. Friedson, this is Lorne Vansickle. I have a cow down with milk fever. She is in the shavings shed. I left her in there because I was sure she would be down by morning. Jess is here. I'll tell him you will be right out."

"Okay, Lorne, I'll take care of it."

"Vansickles have a milk fever," he called out to Bev.

"You can't go, Dad!" Marie blurted out. "What about our program?"

"Milk fevers are emergencies, Honey. If they aren't attended to right away, the cow might die," he answered.

Alice stood up. "Well, the service is only an hour. You could go then."

Bev came out of the bathroom and asked, "Did he say how long she has been down?"

"No, but I am sure she is a heavy milker and it will hit her quite hard. I suppose I could call Jess and ask."

Allan looked up at his dad and said, "It would be nice if you didn't miss our service. We really have worked hard. But if you have to go, I understand."

"You know, Bev," Alton said, "I could go for the children's parts and then skip out. They don't participate in the last half of the service. The senior class is giving the sermon. I could still be at Lorne's in 45 minutes."

"It's your decision. I know the kids would like you to be there."

When the Prodigal Son skit was over, Alton hurried to his Ford and headed out to the Vansickle dairy.

Milk fever, or eclampsia, is a metabolic condition very common in high producing milk cows, occurring within 24 to 48 hours after calving. It is caused by a lack of calcium circulating to the organs and tissues of the body. When a heavy milk producer has her calf, her first instinct is to produce a large amount of milk and deposit it into the udder, which, through selective breeding is large and can hold many pounds of milk. Of course milk is very high in calcium and in order for the cow to produce large quantities, she drains the calcium level from her system. This has a serious affect on the muscles and nervous system and causes paralysis, unconsciousness and a quick death if not treated because the diaphragm becomes paralyzed and the animal cannot breathe.

The treatment is quite simple, and very effective and even quite dramatic, but it has to be given soon after symptoms are visible or the cow may not recover. If treatment is delayed, she could suffer brain damage and never return to normalcy. Calcium, given intravenously, is the treatment of choice and has a high rate of efficacy. A veterinarian slips a needle into the jugular vein and slowly runs the calcium solution into the blood system, replenishing the low calcium count. Within minutes the heart rate returns to normal, the muscles begin to tone up, the respiration picks up and soon the cow is on her feet. By the time the doctor has his equipment cleaned up and put back in his vehicle, the cow is out of danger and ready to join the herd. However if the cow has been sick and down for a long period of time and the veterinarian procrastinates or is negligent, there is a good chance the dairyman will have a dead cow.

Dr. Friedson stopped his car in front of the milking parlor. As he was opening the trunk to get his equipment, Mr. Vansickle stepped out of the back door onto the porch and hollered in a loud, angry voice, "Don't bother to get your stuff; the cow died! Where have you been? I called you over an hour ago. You'll pay for this. She was one of my best cows. I'm going to sue you and you can tell Branberg that too. You're liable for this and you'll hear from my lawyer."

Before Dr. Friedson could say a word, Mr. Vansickle went back in the house and slammed the door behind him. Dr. Friedson stood with his hand on the car door staring at the house. He whispered to himself, "What does he mean, the cow died? She couldn't have died. Maybe he didn't check her to be sure."

He swung the door open, slid into the front seat and gripped the steering wheel. He sat motionless as his heart began to pound, sweat beads formed on his forehead and his hands began to shake. He knew he had made a mistake, he knew he was liable, and he knew he would have to suffer the consequences.

It was only four miles back to the hospital but it seemed like a hundred. Thoughts raced through his head, and they weren't good ones. He knew he shouldn't have waited – milk fevers are always a first priority. Dr. Branberg was going to be terribly upset. Mr. Vansickle would spread the word that Dr. Friedson was negligent, was incompetent and liable for a lawsuit. His whole world was tumbling down on him just because he followed his heart and not his head. He parked behind the hospital and decided not to talk to anyone until he had had a chance to clear his head.

A few questions began popping up in his mind, and some didn't make sense. "First, why was Mr. Vansickle so short with me? He didn't come out to the car. Just stood on the porch and hollered. Most angry farmers take the opportunity to get right in the culprit's face. And he didn't bother to take me out to the shed and show me the dead cow. There had to be proof that the cow died. Second, when Vansickle called, he said the hired man Jess was there to help me if needed. That meant that Jess was working, and if so, why didn't he make the call? Third, Jess would have arrived at the barn at 5:00 a.m. and would have checked on the cow immediately if there was concern that she might go down. If she was still alive, he would have called immediately. Things didn't add up, and maybe I'm not in as much trouble as I first thought."

Was there a possibility that the cow was already dead when Jess looked in on her at 5:00 a.m.? When Mr. Vansickle looked in on her at 10:30 a.m. he probably didn't check her closely, just assumed she was still alive and called the vet to come and treat her. When he checked her an hour later and found her cold, stiff, and dead, he may have realized his mistake and tried to save face. If all this was true, then Dr. Friedson had to formulate a plan and he would have to be a little sneaky for it to be successful.

He drove back to the dairy and instead of driving into the barnyard past the house, he took the service road used by the hay, feed, and milk trucks and parked on the west side of the milk parlor out of sight of the house. He opened the trunk and took out the stainless steel pail, the rubber intravenous tube, a new 16-gauge needle, a pair of nose tongs and a 500ml bottle of calcium gluconate. When he entered the parlor, he waved a hello to Jess and headed directly to the sink and began running hot water into the pail. Jess walked over to him and with a curious look on his face asked, "What are you going to do, Dr. Fried?"

"Lorne called and said you have a milk fever down."

"Well, we did," he replied, "but she died. She was dead when I came to work at five this morning."

"She was already dead when you came at five? Are you sure?" Alton questioned.

"Sure as guns. I kicked her legs and she was stiff as a board. Must have been dead for several hours."

"Was she okay when you left last night?" Dr. Friedson asked.

"Yes, but we suspected she would go down. She gives a hundred pounds a day."

"Then why didn't you look at her later?"

"I offered to," Jess said, shrugging his shoulders,

"But Mr. Vansickle said they were going out to a dinner party and he would check on her when he got home around midnight. He probably had a few drinks and forgot."

"I suspect that's what happened. You are sure she was dead when you came early this morning?" Dr. Friedson wanted to be sure of the time.

"Yeah. I checked her first thing when I got here this morning."

Dr. Friedson asked if he could see the cow, and with Jess's permission he walked to the shavings shed. The legs on the big Holstein were as rigid as a board and she was already beginning to bloat. Dr. Friedson estimated she had been dead for about nine hours, which would put the time of death at around 3:00 a.m. Lorne and his wife probably got home shortly before this and went directly to bed.

Dr. Friedson drove back to hospital feeling much better than he had an hour earlier. He had dodged a bullet, but even though he would be exonerated, he still had to face the fact that he was negligent and under different circumstances it could have been disastrous for him. He had learned a lesson.

The following Wednesday, Mr. Vansickle called the hospital and told Rachel he wanted to talk to both doctors and made an appointment for 3:00 p.m. Dr. Friedson was terribly nervous about what would be said and what might happen, but he had all the facts and was ready to defend his position. He had told the whole story to Dr. Branberg and assured him that there was no liability on the part of himself or Dr. Branberg.

Lorne spoke in a quiet, humble, apologetic voice, explaining that he did not check the cow when he returned from his dinner and assumed she was alive when he made the call to Dr. Friedson. When he found her dead later, he lost his cool and flew off the handle, thinking it was Dr. Friedson's fault for being late. When he found out what had really happened, he felt ashamed and sorry for how he had acted. After talking it over with his wife, they agreed he should apologize and assure both doctors that it was his entire fault, their doctor/client relationship was in good standing and he would be more attentive in the future.

The whole incident could have turned out to be very unpleasant for everyone involved, but because Mr. Vansickle was a gentleman and did the right thing, all was forgiven and forgotten.

THIRTEEN

I t was noon, and Dr. Friedson had stopped at the Broaster for a bowl of soup when another customer at the restaurant approached his table and asked, "You're Dr. Friedson, are you not?"

"Yes, I'm Alton Friedson," he answered, looking up.

"I know this isn't proper, but I have been meaning to call you for some time but just haven't got around to it." The man sat down without being invited, and Alton told himself this could be a long story. Alton just sat and looked at him.

"I have a dog, a Chow, with eye problems. He's had it for years and I have treated it with ointments and drops, which seems to help but it doesn't clear up. The eyes water and matter all the time and he constantly rubs them with his front paws."

Alton swallowed the cracker he was chewing on and asked, "Have you had many Chows?"

"I have two, but the other one is okay. By the way, my name is Harry Coleman; the dog's name is Chan." He extended a rough, chapped hand and gave Alton a short, strong handshake.

"Chows have a history of eye problems, it's hereditary and many bloodlines pass it on in every litter. We see a lot of it in this area. Did you get the dog from someone around here?"

"Yeah, a family I knew up river had a litter and gave me Chan. That has to be ten years now."

"My gosh! He's had the problem for ten years? Have you taken him to a clinic to have the problem corrected?" Alton was taken aback, thinking this poor dog had been suffering for ten years.

"I've seen a couple of docs and they gave me medicine to put in the eyes but, like I said, they didn't seem to help much. I just assumed there wasn't much that could be done. Now he is really bad and I may have to put him down."

"Do you live in town, Mr. Coleman?" Alton asked.

"Yeah, north on 33rd street," he answered.

"Could you bring Chan in to my hospital tomorrow afternoon? I could look at him and see if something can be done. Do you know where my hospital is?"

Harry pushed back his chair and stood up, "It's over here on Westside isn't it? I'll have him there right after lunch. I won't clean the eyes so you can see how bad they are," he pulled his dirty felt hat down over his eyes and left through the back door.

Judging from his attire and rough hands, Alton guessed Mr. Coleman to be a logger. Because of the mountains and thick forests, logging was a big industry in the area and a large number of the local residents depended on the logging and lumber mills for employment. Logging was a tough, backbreaking way to make a living and most of the men who worked in the woods were strong and burly and had a macho way about them. Most of them drove old, beat-up trucks with a couple of rifles strapped to the rear window and four or five spotlights bolted to a three-inch roll bar welded to the frame just behind the cab. It seemed that every one of them had a couple of dogs that spent the majority of their time in the back of the pickup. There was every breed imaginable from Hounds to Dalmatians. The dogs were their pride and joy, and they gave them excellent care.

Harry Coleman walked into the hospital pulling Chan behind him with a short piece of twine. Rachel completed the paperwork, and after directing Harry and Chan into the exam room she hurried to the office and started ragging on Alton about what a mess the dog was.

"For gosh sakes, Dr. Fried, that poor dog hasn't been groomed in years. He has large mats hanging from his ears and belly, straw and sticks are stuck to his coat and he stinks to high heaven. And his eyes are matted shut, he has to be blind. How can a person do that to someone they say is their best friend? Some people make me sick," she said as she stomped off to her desk.

Alton knew even before he saw the dog what the diagnosis was going to be. The condition was hereditary in Chows, and because of their small eyes and loose skin a majority of the breed had the problem to some extent. The condition is called lower lid entropion; the lower lid rolls in toward the eyeball, causing the eye- lashes and skin hair to rub against the cornea resulting in a severe case of conjunctivitis, pannus, and corneal ulceration. It is extremely painful, and if the condition is not corrected, many dogs will go blind at an early age.

"Good afternoon, Harry," Dr. Friedson said as he entered the room. He stood with his back against the desk away from the dog because Chows have a history of being a little unfriendly. "Is Chan friendly or does he not take to strangers too well?"

"You better introduce yourself slowly. When he can't see, he gets jumpy when someone touches him or gets too close. If I hold his head he will be okay," Harry said as he put his arm around Chan's neck and held him by the nose.

After washing the matter from the eyes and examining the lids, Alton concluded that the problem was bilateral entropion with a moderate case of corneal ulceration.

Alton stood back, folded his arms and said, "Well, it is just as I suspected, Harry. Chan has bilateral entropion, meaning the lower lids rub against the cornea of the eyes, causing several problems. Alton rolled Chan's lower eye lids in and out showing Harry the condition and how it causes injury to the eyeball. He explained how ointments and drops would give some relief but would not cure the problem and said corrective surgery was the only permanent solution.

"How much would that cost to have both eyes done?" Harry seemed concerned about the price.

"The procedure is not difficult but time-consuming and exacting because the right amount of skin has to be removed so that the lids are not too tight or too loose. The total price for both eyes would be $80.00. We would keep Chan overnight and send him home the next day with some ointment and you would return in ten days to have the sutures removed. I could do it tomorrow if you want to bring him back in the morning."

"Do I have to pay it all at once?" Harry asked

"That would be preferable, but we can make some payment arrangements. We can help you out because the surgery needs to be done – Chan has suffered enough." Alton was sorry he had used the word suffer as it made Harry look bad, but the dog had to be in pain.

The appointment was made, Dr. Friedson would do the surgery, and Mr. Coleman would make a payment on his bill and take Chan home the following day.

When Mr. Coleman saw Chan with his eyes wide open with no squinting, no tearing, and no sticky matter, he was delighted. "Well, look at you. Do you feel better, Buddy?" Chan rubbed against Harry's legs and wagged his tail and looked up at him as if to thank his master for taking away the irritation and discomfort that he had endured for so long.

"He looks great, Doc. I should have done this long ago. By the way, I am going to pay the whole bill; I get paid this Friday."

Harry was instructed to put the ophthalmic ointment in Chan's eyes three times a day and to bring him back in ten to twelve days to have the stitches taken out. He shook hands with both Alton and Rachel and left expressing how pleased he was and would give a call if there were any problems.

Rachel put Mr. Coleman's card in the POP file for a call-back in three days, which she did, but after several tries she was unable to get an answer. After several days of trying she finally gave up, assuming he was in the woods and unable to answer the phone.

Harry Coleman never called the hospital and didn't bring Chan in to have the sutures removed from the lower lids. Alton just assumed that everything had turned out satisfactorily and that the case was closed. Chan's card was removed from the POP rack and placed in the permanent file.

It was six weeks since Dr. Friedson had done the surgery on Chan's eyes, and as he was going through the daily mail he noticed a letter with a return address from the Washington State Board of Governors. Thinking it was an announcement or special request, he carelessly ripped it open and quickly scanned the contents. He was surprised when he saw his name underlined and even more surprised when he read that he had been reported for malpractice.

The official letter read that a complaint had been filed against him, Doctor Alton Friedson, State License Number 1233, by a mister Harry Coleman, for performing surgery on his ten-year-old black chow named Chan, without the owner's permission. The complaint stated that Mr. Coleman had brought his dog into the Valley Veterinary Hospital for an examination because his eyes were bothering him. It stated that Dr. Alton Friedson looked at the dog and suggested that Mr. Coleman bring the dog back the next morning. As requested, Mr. Coleman dropped Chan off at the hospital and went to work. When he returned to pick up the dog, he was not only surprised but extremely upset that surgery had been performed without his permission. The complaint stated that Mr. Coleman was under the impression that the condition of the eyes was to be evaluated and a suitable treatment would be decided after a consultation.

The letter requested Dr. Friedson submit a written response and a hearing would be scheduled after the Board had studied the case and determined if the complaint was legitimate.

Both Dr. Friedson and Dr. Branberg were extremely concerned about the complaint because it was a black mark against the reputation of the hospital, and they were equally disappointed in Mr. Coleman for making such an accusation after the doctors had given his dog such excellent care. There had to be an underlying reason for him to take such drastic action but at the time, no one could put their finger on it.

Dr. Friedson returned a letter to the Board of Governors explaining the events leading up to Mr. Coleman's visit to the veterinary hospital, the events the day of the surgery, and how pleased Mr. Coleman was when he picked the dog up as scheduled. Mr. Coleman had showed no evidence of surprise that surgery had been done and had expressed his gratitude for what had been done to correct the long-standing problem. He thought the price for treatment was fair, and he paid the bill in full.

Dr. Friedson closed the letter by requesting he receive a copy of the original complaint as written by Mr. Harry Coleman.

Alton desperately wanted to contact Harry and get a first hand explanation for the complaint, but after many tries it was obvious it wasn't going to happen because when Coleman realized who was calling, he would hang up the phone. The only recourse was to stop by his house and catch him at home.

The first time Alton stopped at the house on north 33rd Street, a pickup was in the driveway, but no one answered the door and Alton could hear no noise coming from inside the house. If Harry was home, he had no intention of speaking with Dr. Friedson. On his second trip to the house the truck was gone and there was no answer at the door but as he turned to leave, there was a noise in the back yard and suddenly two dogs came running around the corner of the house and jumped against the chain link fence. Alton immediately recognized the black Chow and walked over and called his name. As Chan stood with his paws against the fence, Alton had a good look at the dog's face. The hair had grown back over the incisions and the eyes were wide open with no watering and no sign of irritation. Alton was totally confused as he stood and watched what appeared to be two normal, happy dogs.

It was obvious to Alton as he read the letter of complaint received from the Board of Governors that it was not written by Harry Coleman. The style, the language, the grammar and use of medical terms were beyond Coleman's capability so he would have to have had professional help. What was his motive, and who would assist him in such a scheme without checking on the facts so as not to get into an embarrassing situation? Alton assumed the help came from a veterinarian because Coleman's complaint stated that he was told the surgery wasn't necessary and that the ointment prescribed following the surgery was harmful to the dog's eyes.

Two weeks passed before Dr. Friedson heard from the State. He was to report to the front desk of the State Veterinary Medical Association building and be prepared to defend his case against the complaint submitted by Mr. Harry Coleman. The letter said he could bring any evidence to support his case and any witnesses who would be willing to be sworn in.

The hearing room was set up quite simply with two tables at one end and a dozen chairs facing the tables. He didn't recognize any of the men seated at the tables but recalled hearing and reading their names when they were introduced as members of the State Board of Governors.

Mr. Coleman was introduced as the complainant and was

asked to present his case by reading the letter of complaint. He emphasized the point that the surgery was done without his permission and certainly would not have approved the drastic surgery if it was suggested because he didn't think it was necessary. He added that another veterinarian told him that considerable damage had been done to the corneas of the eyes because Dr. Friedson had prescribed a steroid ointment for aftercare. When asked if he was unhappy with the whole incident, Mr. Coleman answered emphatically that he had endured a great amount of anxiety and grief and unnecessary expense because of the unprofessional way the case was handled, and that Dr. Friedson should be properly reprimanded.

Alton presented his side of the case by stating everything exactly the way it happened. He was quite confident in his presentation until the end, when one board member asked him plain and clear if he had evidence of a written statement that Mr. Coleman had authorized the surgery. Alton had a sinking feeling when he truthfully answered it was given orally but not in writing.

The members confided for a few minutes, then the presiding member stood and announced the case was closed. He thanked both parties for participating and said each would receive a copy of the verdict in two weeks.

Dr. Friedson was furious. He felt empty. He felt he wasn't given the time or the opportunity to fully explain the situation, to present his hospital procedure or to tell how the dog was suffering when he was brought into the clinic. He wanted to tell how comfortable and happy Chan was when he saw him in the yard. He wanted to ask about the other veterinarian and how he got involved. He wanted and expected a lengthy question and answer period to prove he had done nothing wrong and had handled the situation both professionally and as requested. He had a lot of questions but no opportunity to ask them. He was escorted out of the room, and when he got to the reception area Harry Coleman was nowhere to be seen.

The follow-up letter from the Board of Governors was short and to the point. Dr. Alton Friedson was guilty of performing major surgery on a client's dog without written permission, causing undue stress, anxiety and hardship on the client and his dog. The penalty was fourfold.

1.   Dr. Friedson would pay a penalty of $1800.00 to the State Veterinary Medical Association.

2.   Dr. Friedson would attend twenty hours of continuous education on ophthalmology pertaining to the dog.

3.   Dr. Friedson would be on medical probation for two years.

4.   Dr. Friedson would reimburse Mr. Coleman for any and all expenses pertaining to the case at hand and make retribution for any physical or mental damage done to the complainant due to Dr. Friedson's incompetence.

As the three of them, Dr. Friedson, Dr. Branberg and Rachel read the letter over and over again, they could not believe the verdict or the severity of the penalty.

Rachel began to cry and shouted, "It is totally unfair! The man is a liar and a cheat! The board didn't give you a chance!"

"Well, what is done is done." Alton said. "We all know we did the right thing and the dog doesn't have to suffer."

"That doesn't make it right," she cried, "there isn't a more caring, compassionate, and dedicated doctor in the whole state than you, Dr. Fried and you shouldn't be accused of something like this. I know that some other vet has it in for you, for some ungodly reason, and he used this situation to get to you. I know it."

Dr. Branberg sat on the edge of his desk with his arms folded across his chest. "We know in our hearts what is right and what is wrong. Alton, we will pay the fine, you will enroll in the classes, and we won't worry about the probation. If Mr. Coleman submits a bill for expenses, we will pay it, and then go on about our business. We are not going to fret or dwell upon what might have been or who did what. Even though we feel we did nothing wrong, we did make a mistake and we are going to learn from it. From now on we get written permission for all major procedures done not only in the hospital but on the farms. I will have a form printed."

Once a month the Washington State Veterinary Medical Association publishes a paper that is circulated to all the veterinarians who are members and in good standing. The month following the Coleman incident there was a report in the paper from the Board of Governors including the judgment against Dr. Friedson. During the week following the distribution there were many calls to the Valley Veterinary Hospital from friends and associates asking questions about the case, expressing concerns and saying how Dr. Friedson had been unjustly wronged. Most of the callers were sympathetic and encouraged the doctors not to worry about it because the veterinary profession considered the Valley Veterinary Hospital to be a first- class practice and Dr. Friedson was known for his professionalism as a veterinarian.

FOURTEEN

I f a tally were kept on all the calls that came in between midnight and 3:00 a.m., Dr. Friedson could tell you that horse emergencies outnumber all other animals for after-hour calls.

The phone rang for what he thought was the second time and when he looked at the clock and saw it was 1:15 a.m., he knew it was a horse client calling. His suspicions were verified when he recognized Donna Hoople's voice.

"We just got back from the farewell party for John and Joan, and when I checked the horses I found a mess. Pride has torn her chest open. It looks like a barbwire cut. She must have gotten scared by something and run into the fence because the wire is down and Josie is not in the corral. I don't know why Pride didn't go too but she is standing quietly by the shed."

"Is she bleeding badly?" was Alton's first question.

"I really don't know. I didn't take a close look. It was dark and I wanted to call you right away."

"Get a light and if you see blood spurting or running down her legs, pack the wound with a clean towel and put pressure on it. Don't let her move. Keep her quiet and I'll be there in half an hour."

The Hooples lived ten miles up the south side of the Skagit River on a small ranch where they raised quarter horses. They were thinking of getting into the thoroughbred business and had just bought their first quality mare. They had already reserved a stud breeding and planned to take her to the stud farm after the first of the year. Alton was glad that it wasn't this mare that was injured.

Most everything on the Hoople farm was new, and there was always a project waiting to be completed. Martin and Donna had lived on a small plot of ground just north of Sedro Woolley where they kept two quarter horses in a small shed with a wooden corral and no pasture. Their dream was to own a ranch up-river near Hamilton with plenty of room for a big barn and grassy fields for the horses to romp and play in. When they found this twenty acre place, it was exactly what they wanted. It was situated on high ground with open fields sloping down to some flat lands along the Skagit River. There were a few acres of cedar trees mixed in with alder and maple.

They moved into a modular home and started the construction of a ten box stall barn with covered hay storage and a walled-in bin for dry shavings. Immediate future plans call for a training corral and a gyp ring. Further down the road they plan to put in all wooden fences with sturdy gates and black stain paint.

As he drove to the farm Alton did what he has done many, many times - visualize the extent of the injury according to the type of accident and pertinent information gained from the client, then plan a regiment of surgery and treatment. This one would be rather routine because Donna was not in a panic and most wire cuts on the upper body of a horse were not too serious. First he would control any persistent bleeding, debride tags of loose tissue and skin, and wash the wound with disinfectant soap. Most barbwire cuts are so jagged and ripped that suturing is ineffective and a waste of time. The call itself would take only about twenty to thirty minutes but he would be invited in for a late cup of coffee so he probably wouldn't get home till close to 3:30.

To his surprise, the situation changed in a hurry as soon as he drove into the yard. Donna hurried to the car, crying, "O God,

Dr. Fried, it's terrible; much worse than I thought. I think we will have to put her down. Her legs are practically gone!"

"Did you find Josie?" he asked

"No, not yet. Martin thinks she headed for the river. There is some green grass down there."

"Were they the only two in the corral when this happened?"

"Thank goodness I listened to Martin. I wanted to keep them all out tonight, but he insisted we put the others in because it looked like rain and the corral would get too muddy."

"You said she's standing by the shed. I'll need a good light and a bucket of hot water. Did you have to stop any bleeding?" he asked.

"I couldn't look at it to see. I nearly fainted," she replied in a whisper.

She went to the house, and as Dr. Friedson walked around the barn to the back shed he wondered why Pride would remain up by the shed when Josie ran off to the river. Normally they would stay together. In a few minutes he was to receive his answer.

Alton was a strong person and had seen many gruesome sights during his time in practice, but this was the worst wire cut he had been called to treat. When he looked at it he nearly threw up, not from the sight of the blood and torn tissues but from the thought of the whole situation. The fright and pain of the horse, the massive destruction of tissue, and the anguish and anxiety of the owners was overwhelming. He could hear himself murmuring, "I don't know what to do. Where do I begin?" Donna stood with her arms folded, one hand covering her mouth as she watched the "master healer", the one who was supposed to cure all ills and make everything better, helplessly shaking his head.

To clear his mind, Alton decided to start from the beginning. Not that it would help with the treatment, but it would give him time to think. Martin had returned with Josie and put her in the barn; thankfully there was not a mark on her. The three of them walked the corral, following the wire and trying to piece together what might have happened. There were two strands that had been twisted together. The most obvious sign was that there was skin and meat on every barb of both wires for at least 150 feet. Obviously Pride had run into the wires and as she ran along them the barbs acted like a saw and tore the skin, muscles and vessels from the bone. After a short discussion they came to a unanimous conclusion.

Something, possibly a deer or coyote, scared the horses and ran them into the fence. Pride was probably on the inside with Josie pressing her against the wires which tore up her legs until the wire broke. Josie kept running down to the river but Pride couldn't follow because with her muscles and nerves severed she couldn't move her front legs.

Returning to the horse, Alton had decided what to do. There was the question of putting Pride to sleep, but that was quickly dismissed when Alton explained the different scenarios, all of which were acceptable to the Hooples. After a considerable length of time the circulation would re-establish itself and the nerves and tendons could possibly reconnect, but muscles don't regenerate so scar tissue would fill in where the muscle would normally be. This would prevent the legs from extending normally so her stride would be hindered and she would never be a trail horse, endurance horse or cattle cutter. But because of her breeding, she could make an excellent brood mare and produce valuable foals. Her sire was McLeo Bars so a foal by a prominent stud could be quite valuable. The decision was to let the legs heal as well as possible, then go from there.

Alton decided not to wash or clean the wounds because solid clots had formed on the major vessels and if disturbed could cause some serious bleeding. A matrix of platelets, serum, and blood cells had formed deep in the wounds, which would enhance the healing process. The primary concerns were to keep the tissues from drying out, prevent infection and keep the horse confined to a small area to limit movement.

After going down the list of possible treatments, Alton decided to use aloe vera jelly because of its healing powers, moisturizing effect, antibacterial properties and relatively inexpensive cost. He soaked cotton in the jelly and laid it carefully into the wounds, holding it in place with a snug bandage. He gave Pride a heavy dose of penicillin and a tetanus booster, though tetanus was not a big concern because the clostridium tetani is basically an anaerobe and usually doesn't like to grow in large open wounds. After the wounds were attended to, the next problem was how to get Pride back to the barn and into a small stall. According to Alton there was only one way, and it was going to be hard and slow. They would have to lift and move her front legs for her, one at a time. To her credit, Pride was cooperative and with Donna leading and Martin lifting and moving the left leg and Alton doing the same to the right leg, they were able to get her settled into a clean, warm stall. Being 10x10 it was not as small as Alton would have liked, but it was the best they had.

His instructions to the Hooples were to go to the health food store and pick up all the aloe vera jelly they had; it was going to take a lot. They agreed to change the dressing once a day and keep the horse as inactive as possible since excessive movement would delay the healing process. If he didn't hear from them, Alton would return in a week to see how things were going.

Donna couldn't thank him enough. She was much relieved and was all hugs and smiles although her heart was aching. Alton took a rain check on the coffee as it was already 4:00 a.m. and he knew he had early morning calls. He settled into the truck and heaved a long sigh as if to say, "Just another night in the life of an equine veterinarian."

FIFTEEN

C alls for veterinary service come from many different people and in many different ways. Most, of course, come by telephone when a client calls to make an appointment for the doctor to make a farm call, or a house call, or requests a time to bring their pet into the hospital. Some clients drop into the hospital to talk to one of the doctors about a problem and end up making an appointment. It often happen that Dr. Friedson or Dr. Branberg ran into a person at a business in town, and during their conversation an appointment would be made to look at an animal that hadn't been feeling well for a few days. Often appointments are made by clients encountered at a restaurant, standing in line to get into a movie, sitting in the waiting room at the medical center, or going out the door after church. Dr. Friedson could recall dozens of veterinary calls made to farms because of encounters with clients at odd hours at different places.

The strangest came one morning when Rachel had taken the monthly finance sheets to the accountant and Alton was alone in the clinic. Foster, the mailman, walked in and, in his usual loud, cheery voice said, "I see they finally caught up with you, Dr. Fried. I knew it was just a matter of time." Foster was a familiar fixture on the west side of town because he was the only mail carrier people had known for many years. Alton judged him to be in his late fifties, but he stepped lively along his route, had a wave and a greeting to everyone he met and had a great sense of humor which he enjoyed using at the drop of a hat.

He slapped an envelope on the counter and pointed to the

green label pasted to the left side of the envelope just under the return address that said Barnes and Bugle, Attorneys at Law.

"Just sign your freedom away on the line there, Mr. Jailbird. I suppose I could be a nice guy and visit you now and then." He laughed as he tore off the label and put it in his bag. I know those lawyers over there in Sedro Woolley, they're tough."

"Yeah, come and see me, Joker. Maybe we could play some chess or gin. Bring the cake with the goodies in I," Alton waved at him.

"See ya, Doc."

Alton had never received a letter from a lawyer's office and was hesitant to open it. The one good sign was that it was thin, which may mean that it didn't contain a lot of bad news. Maybe it was an invitation to an investment meeting or banquet to raise money for a charity. He tore open the end, blew on the edges to separate them, reached inside and pulled out the one page letter. In bold letters the letterhead read Barnes and Bugle, Attorneys at Law, with a street address in Sedro Woolley. He unfolded the letter and as he began to read he gave a sigh of relief because he immediately realized it was nothing involving him or the practice. It was a plea for help. Jerry and Arlene Rucker, a small ranch family, were suing Joan Retling, a veterinarian, for lack of competence, knowledge and skill. The lawyers were representing the couple in the suit and were writing Dr. Friedson asking him to testify as a professional witness. The letter was a courtesy request hoping he would volunteer his services because, according to the attorneys, Alton was the most qualified equine veterinarian in the area for the case at hand, and they wanted the best. If he declined to appear voluntarily, they would subpoena him to take the stand.

Alton knew immediately that he was between a rock and a hard place; he had done some business with the Rucker family and was good friends with Dr. Retling. Even before he read the details of the suit, he knew it was a no-win situation for him regardless of how it turned out.

Several days after requesting a copy of the Rucker's deposition, he received a letter from the law firm describing the events as told by Mrs. Rucker.

On April 10th Arlene Rucker had called Dr. Retling to examine a sore foot on one of her beef cows and castrate one of their spring calves. Joan Retling was a young veterinarian in her middle thirties who operated a large animal mobile practice, driving from farm to farm in her elaborately equipped custom-built van. She didn't advertise her small animal services but did vaccinate and do minor surgeries on dogs and cats when on the farms. Her expertise was in beef cattle, hogs, sheep and goats but she was slowly expanding her practice into ponies and horses. Although she was a competent and well-respected veterinarian, Dr. Friedson had heard reports of some of her equine cases that hadn't turned out for the best. Twice she had called him to ask his advice on a procedure she was not familiar with.

Dr. Retling had been cleaning her equipment after doctoring the cow's foot and castrating the calf, when Mrs. Rucker asked her if she had time to examine a mare that was due to foal within the week.

Dr. Friedson read the deposition as given by Mrs. Rucker.

Mrs. Rucker, "Dr. Retling was cleaning her equipment and didn't seem to be in a hurry to leave, so I asked her if she would have time to check a mare that was scheduled to foal in a few days. She said she would be glad to do it. She finished her cleaning, took a leather kit from her van and asked where the mare was. I led her to the horse barn and walked to the stall where Mistymorning was standing quietly with her head in the corner of the large, straw-bedded foaling stall."

Mr. Barnes, "What did Dr. Retling say when she saw the mare?"

Mrs. Rucker, "She asked if the mare had been showing any signs of labor or discomfort. I told her not that I had noticed."

Mr. Barnes, "Please tell us what happened next."

Mrs. Rucker, "I put a halter on Mist and Dr. Retling entered the stall and did a quick exam, feeling her udder and looking under her tail. She then did a rectal palpation to check the status and position of the foal. After a few minutes she got a puzzled look on her face, which I took to mean there may be a problem."

Mr. Barnes, "Did she say anything to indicate there was a problem?"

Mrs. Rucker, "She said the foal was high in the birth canal but she suspected there may be a problem with the cervix. It seemed larger than it should be. She said she needed to do a vaginal exam. She put on a clean glove and inserted her arm into the vagina. After a few minutes she withdrew her arm and said she found nothing abnormal but was still confused about the cervix. She again inserted her arm into the rectum and after only a few seconds said, "Just as I suspected. We have a serious situation. The mare has a twisted uterus."

Mr. Barnes, "Excuse me. Did she say this with a lot of assurance or was she a little hesitant?"

Mrs. Rucker, "She was confident about the condition but she was hesitant about what to do about it. She said the foal couldn't be born unless the condition was corrected and there were only two possibilities; untwist the uterus manually or do a caesarian. At this point I was becoming very concerned and quite worried."

Mr. Barnes, "At this point did you start asking questions?"

Mrs. Rucker, "I asked a lot of questions. How did this happen? Why wasn't the mare in pain?" How long could this have been this way? How long could the foal live? She said the most common cause was from the mare rolling vigorously, revolving the body around the uterus and causing it to twist just anterior to the cervix. It usually doesn't cause pain even though it ties the uterus shut so the foal can't be expelled. She explained that when the mare goes into labor, the uterus will contract but the foal is trapped inside. Two things can happen, together or separately. The uterus can rupture causing the foal to die, or the umbilical cord can break causing the foal to suffocate.

Mr. Barnes, "Did you ask her what she would recommend?"

Mrs. Rucker, "I asked her what we should do and how much time we had."

Mr. Barnes, "What did she say? It is important that you give us exactly what she said."

Mrs. Rucker, "Well I can't recite the exact word for word, but she indicated that a cesarean was the best approach and it had to be done immediately. This really set me back because I couldn't understand the urgency. Mistymorning seemed very relaxed and comfortable and not the least bit in labor. I questioned her decision but she said according to the signs Mist was going to go into labor real soon so the surgery had to be done right away."

Mr. Barnes, "Did you consent to her request?"

Mrs. Rucker, "I said I would like to get a second opinion. Maybe call Dr. Friedson or at least call an equine hospital and get an appointment for the surgery. She said there wasn't time and that she would have to perform the caesarian right there in the stall."

Mr. Barnes, "Were you okay with that?"

Mrs. Rucker, "Heavens no. I was confused, scared and had a dozen questions. Everything was happening so fast and I couldn't understand it. My husband was away on a trip and I wasn't used to making on-the-spot, serious decisions concerning the animals."

Mr. Barnes, "What did you ask her?"

Mrs. Rucker, "I asked her if she had performed a caesarian on a mare before and she said no but it was not much different than on a cow and she had done several of those. I also suggested that we get some help but she said it wasn't necessary, but if it made me feel better she would call her neighbor friend and she could assist. She came to help but she was inexperienced and didn't contribute much."

Mr. Barnes, "Please tell us about the surgery and what happened to the mare and foal."

Mrs. Rucker, "Dr. Retling set up her equipment while I bedded the stall with clean straw and carried in three pails of hot water. She gave Mistymorning an anesthetic by injecting a solution into her jugular vein, and within seconds she went down hard with a little struggle. We rolled her over on to her back and propped her up with hay bales. Dr. Retling tied a bottle of anesthetic to one of the bars along the stall partition and set it to slowly drip during the surgery."

Mr. Barnes, "How were you feeling at this point?"

Mrs. Rucker, "I still questioned whether the surgery was necessary at this time and if we were doing the right thing. I told her I was nervous and unsure about the whole situation, but she assured me it was going to be alright. After scrubbing and disinfecting the lower belly she made a large incision along the midline she spread the opening and declared, 'there folks, is the uterus. Now all we have to do is get that little baby horse out of there.' Well, let me tell you, it was a mess and a struggle. She and her friend couldn't lift the foal out, being slippery and heavy and all so we had to remove the hay bales and roll the mare on her side. In doing so the intestines began pushing out onto the straw, getting dirty and contaminated. Dr Retling began pushing them back and stuffing towels in the belly. She told me to use my hands and arms to try and keep the innards from rolling out while she attended to the foal. She pulled the foal out onto the floor, cleaned the mucous from its nose and heaved a sigh of relief when it took a deep gasp and began to breathe."

Mr. Barnes, "Did you relax a little when the foal appeared to be alright?"

Mrs. Rucker, "Well yes, but my arms were getting tired and I had some concerns about Misty. She had a long incision in her belly and I didn't see how she was going to nurse her baby. In fact there was little to no milk in her udder and she was going to be sore. We were sitting back on our heels resting when the so-called assistant quietly said, "You know, Joan, I haven't seen the mare take a breath for some time; she must be really deep." Dr. Retling looked at Misty's head, then up to the IV bottle then, mostly to herself said, "Oh, no!" and quickly jumped up. The mare had no eye reflex, her membranes were dark blue, and there was no pulse. She was dead."

Mr. Barnes, "Did she try to revive her?"

Mrs. Rucker, "No. She evidently had been dead for several minutes. She had received an overdose of anesthetic. During the stress of getting the foal out, Dr. Retling had forgotten to monitor the anesthetic drip and was supposed to add only a small amount of the anesthetic as she needed it, not the whole bottle."

Mr. Barnes, "Did she admit to the overdose?"

Mrs. Rucker, "Not really. She alluded to the fact that under normal circumstances a mare Misty's size could tolerate that much drug but because of the stress and the pain, the combination of events was too much for her."

Mr. Barnes, "So after acknowledging that the mare was dead and beyond help, what did she do next?"

Mrs. Rucker, "She attended to the foal, treating the navel, giving an antibiotic, and wiping her down to dry her off. She then stood up and said, 'Well, this is what we have to do. I will call the dead animal service to come and pick up the mare, then I will take the baby home with me. She will need IV fluids, will have to be taught how to nurse a bottle and will need some extra special care several hours a day. I don't think you can do it, Arlene, so I will take over for you.' I think I went into another state of shock."

Mr. Barnes, "Did she take the foal and leave?"

Mrs. Rucker, "Yes, she bundled the filly up, put it in her truck, and while she was washing up she apologized profusely, saying she was extremely sorry but things like this happen and at least I had a live filly, which probably wouldn't have happened without the surgery. She said she would call Morley's Dead Animal Service and would let me know later how the filly was doing. She drove off leaving me standing in the yard trying to sort out the details of just exactly what had happened in the past hour."

Mr. Barnes, "You said you are filing damages for the loss of your mare and her foal. What happened next?"

Mrs. Rucker, "I didn't hear from Dr. Retling for two days, and she didn't return my calls. Then on the third day she called and said she was terribly sorry but the filly died. She said the foal wouldn't take the bottle so she became dehydrated, developed pneumonia due to the drenching procedure, developed diarrhea, kept getting weaker and died. She never got to her feet."

Mr. Barnes, "Okay. I think we have heard enough of the details. One last question. I want you to think carefully about this. Do you honestly and truly feel that Dr. Joan Retling was wrong in her diagnosis, negligent in her surgical procedures, without proper facilities to care for the foal and because of these inadequacies she responsible for the death of your mare Mistymorning and her newborn foal? And if so, why?"

Mrs. Rucker, "I have consulted with the equine specialists at the Washington State Veterinary College and talked to several Equine Veterinarians and they all emphatically agree that the mare and foal had little to no chance of survival considering the circumstances, the procedures performed, the inadequate facilities, and the lack of experience of both the doctor and assistant. They all questioned that the mare didn't appear to be close to labor, they questioned the diagnosis of the twisted uterus. They all stated that few mares recover from a midline caesarian in hospitals and hardly ever when the surgery is performed in a barn. Their consensus was that a foal that won't nurse a proxy mare or bottle will almost always die. Two of the doctors questioned the diagnosis because uterine torsion in a mare is extremely rare.

Mr. Barnes, "This concludes the deposition."

From overhearing conversations at the local coffee shops and talking to a few clients, Alton knew that the Ruckers had lost a pregnant mare but he didn't know the circumstances or the details of the case until after reading the deposition. Without further information or talking to Arlene or the attorneys, Alton knew that if what Mrs. Rucker said was true, then in his own mind the Ruckers would win the suit. Even though Dr. Retling did what she thought was best, she ended up losing the mare and foal. As much as he hated to injure or even possibly destroy a colleague's reputation, such an error in judgment could not be let go. He would write a letter to Barnes and Bugle stating he would willingly take the stand and testify as a professional witness for the prosecution.

SIXTEEN

D r. Friedson was called to take the stand on trial day seven. He was introduced as a professional witness as an equine practitioner testifying for the prosecution. The first half hour was spent questioning his credentials as a professional witness and when all participating attorneys were satisfied; Alton placed his hand on the Bible and swore to tell the truth, the whole truth and nothing but the truth.

Mr. Barnes "In your professional opinion, Dr. Friedson, is there a good possibility that Mrs. Rucker's mare Mistymorning was not in labor when Dr. Joan Retling examined her state of pregnancy?"

Dr. Friedson "I strongly doubt if the mare was in labor at the time, and for several reasons:

Number 1. The number of days of the gestation period. A thoroughbred mare's gestation period is 327 days. According to Mistymorning's breeding chart she was bred twice, May 21 and 23, making her expected due date to be April 14. According to Mrs. Rucker's veterinary billing records, Dr. Retling examined the mare on March 30, which is 15 days prior to the earliest due date. Mares seldom foal early. If they miss the due date they are almost consistently late.

Number 2. According to Mrs. Rucker, the mare showed no sign of coming into her milk. Ten to twelve days prior to foaling, a mare's udder will begin to swell and small beads of wax collect on the end of the teats. This is called waxing. If this waxing isn't present, then labor is probably at least two weeks away.

Number 3. The quiet and the restful attitude and demeanor of the mare at the time of the examination. Just prior to and during labor the mare becomes restless, agitated, will go off her feed and often wan to be left alone. Mrs. Rucker will testify that Mistymorning showed none of these symptoms."

Mr. Barnes "So, to the best of your knowledge and what you know, you would state that at the time Mistymorning was examined she was not in labor and probably several days away from foaling?"

Dr. Friedson "Yes."

Mr. Barnes "Dr. Friedson, in your professional opinion and from what you know about this case, do you think the mare in question had a torsion or twist in the uterus at the time Dr. Retling examined the uterus? Please justify your answer."

Dr. Friedson "No! But Dr. Retling was correct in telling Mrs. Rucker that if there was a uterine torsion then it should be treated as an emergency to prevent injury or death to the foal. I doubt if the uterus was twisted. A volvulus, torsion or intussusceptions or anything that affects a smooth muscle organ in a human or animal is extremely painful. With a twisted stomach, intestine, colon or uterus, a horse would be sweating, down and rolling, kicking at the abdomen, have flared nostrils, rapid breathing and be reluctant to move. If one or more of these symptoms were visible, Mrs. Rucker would have known it."

Mr. Barnes "What are the causes for uterine torsion and how does one diagnose the condition?"

Dr. Friedson "Lying on the ground and violently rolling from side to side is the only cause that I am familiar with, and to be truthful I have never seen or diagnosed the condition in all my years working with horses as a veterinarian and as an owner. Mares heavy in foal don't lie down much and they seldom roll unless they are in pain, such as with colic. A term foal can weigh ninety pounds, making it difficult for a mare to do much rolling.

Diagnosis can be difficult because the condition is often confused with intestinal colic. It can elicit similar symptoms, and veterinarians will usually treat the mare for colic. When the mare doesn't respond to treatment, then further examination is necessary. Rectal palpation is necessary to digitally feel the twisted tissue, which can be anterior or posterior to the cervix. It would take an experienced veterinarian to locate and recognize the condition and then know how to correct it."

When Mr. Barnes asked Dr. Friedson if he thought Dr. Retling had the knowledge and experience to make a correct diagnosis, the defense attorney objected and the judge sustained.

Mr. Barnes "Concerning the surgery, do horses usually recover from extensive abdominal surgery or do they often develop complications?"

Dr. Friedson "Horses are extremely sensitive to peritonitis, which is acute inflammation of the abdomen and its contents. In an advanced case, most horses die. Because of this, it is rare that a veterinarian will attempt any surgery involving opening the abdomen unless it is performed in a well-equipped and well-staffed equine hospital. Making a long midline abdominal incision on a 1000-pound horse on the floor in a barn without proper equipment and experienced assistance is using poor judgment and inviting some serious trouble."

Mr. Barnes "Would you perform abdominal surgery on a horse on a farm, in a non-sterile environment, if the situation presented itself?"

Dr. Friedson "The situation has presented itself several times and I have always opted to transport the horse to the nearest equine hospital, which from here is only 65 miles."

Mr. Barnes "In your opinion, under the circumstances, could the foal have been saved?"

Dr. Friedson "I doubt it. Being two weeks premature, the sucking reflex would be too weak and with the mare not having come into her milk there would be no colostrums to give the foal the necessary antibodies for the immune system. The foal would require around-the-clock attention from experienced personnel with special equipment and supplies. Even in equine hospitals such foals rarely make it and if they do they have a poor start."

Mr. Barnes "So, let's summarize. From the deposition you read given by Mrs. Rucker, the testimony you have heard here in the court room, and from your experience as an equine veterinarian, do you think the mare in question, Mistymorning, was in labor or close to labor when Dr. Retling examined her?"

Dr. Friedson "No, I don't."

Mr. Barnes "Do you think the mare had a twisted uterus when Dr. Retling examined her?"

Dr. Friedson "No, I don't."

Mr. Barnes "Do you think it is wise and in good judgment to perform abdominal surgery on an adult horse anywhere but in a large animal hospital?"

Dr. Friedson "No, I don't."

Mr. Barnes "Is saving a premature foal without adequate facilities, supplies and experienced personnel very successful?"

Dr. Friedson "Not usually."

The defense attorneys questioned Alton on his knowledge and experience, often using the terms "isn't it possible" and "isn't it reasonable to assume." Alton stuck to his testimony, which wasn't too difficult because Dr. Retling's case was quite weak and her defense had no solid witnesses to stand up for her.

The trial lasted for five days and the jury came back with a guilty verdict. Alton wasn't real proud of what he had done but he had satisfaction in knowing that justice had been served. He had mixed feelings about jeopardizing Dr. Retling's career but when one makes a hasty, foolish mistake, one must accept the consequences.

The court awarded the Ruckers $176,000: $22,000 for the mare, and $10,000 for each foal she would probably have had for the next ten years, and $34,000 for attorney's fees and court costs. The Ruckers asked for no compensation for grief, mental anxiety, or any other frivolous claim. They were satisfied to cover their financial losses. They wished no long-lasting ill effects on Dr. Retling.

SEVENTEEN

D r. Friedson was in the kennel ward wrapping adhesive tape around a splint that had been applied to stabilize the fractured femur on a German Shepherd. It was a walking splint but the dog was so heavy the tape stretched and the rods and tape had to be tightened every day. An intramedullary pin or Kirshner apparatus would have been more effective, but the bone was so shattered these devices would not have worked. The adaptable Shroeder-Thomas splint was a cumbersome but effective device for healing fractured leg bones.

He had the dog on the floor with its leg propped up on his knee when Rachel poked her head through the door and told him not to leave the hospital because an injured dog was on its way in.

"Mrs. Martin from the Alger Grocery called and said her dog had been run over and needed immediate attention."

"The Doxi or the Healer?" he asked without looking up.

"She didn't say. Just that a car had run over him and skinned his back. She'll be here in twenty minutes."

Mrs. Martin, along with her two young daughters, ran a small grocery and variety store in the little community of Alger. They catered mostly to the local residents and nearby farmers. The three of them lived in an apartment in the back of the store, which was convenient for their customers because when the store was closed they could knock on the door when they needed something that absolutely couldn't wait until morning. The Martins had two dogs that were permanent fixtures in the front of the store and their sole purpose in life was to greet the patrons and beg for a handout.

Benny, the Australian Blue Healer, was not overly friendly but he quickly jumped to his feet and wagged his stumpy tail when people called him by name and offered a quick pat on the head. His favorite resting area was under the front counter, where he had an unobstructed view of the front door and easy pickings if a tidbit fell off the counter and on to the floor.

Schultz, the Dachshund, was lazy, overweight and a worry to everyone who drove up to the front of the store. He loved to lie on the warm pavement near the front door and wouldn't move for anyone or anything. If he did, it was always in the wrong direction and cars had to brake or swerve to avoid hitting him. Everyone knew he was an accident just waiting to happen.

Alton stopped at the store many times a month because it was on his way to many of his clients. It was a quick in-and-out at lunch time for a cup of coffee or a hotdog and a bag of chips. When pulling up, he made a point to locate Schultz and park far enough away to avoid any surprises. When leaving the store he would stand in the doorway with his hand on the screen and shout back to Mrs. Martin, "I'll see you and that wiener dog in my clinic one of these days. I guarantee it!"

Mrs. Martin and her younger daughter came through the front door carrying Schultz in a blood- stained army blanket. It was obvious they both had been crying but they were calm and rational assuring each other that even though Schultz was badly injured, he was not going to die.

The daughter gently laid the dog on the exam table, and when she unwrapped the blanket Dr. Friedson was pleasantly surprised because Schultz seemed bright, alert and in very little pain. There didn't appear to be any obvious serious injuries.

He looked at Mrs. Martin and asked, "What seems to be the problem here?"

She stepped back and with a bloody finger pointed to his back and half shouted, "Well, look at his back – the skin!"

Then Dr. Friedson noticed it. A fold of skin at the back of the head had been turned under and there were streaks of blood along the belly wall. He reached down and picking up the edge of the skin, and as he began pulling it away from the muscles along the back, all hell broke loose.

Mrs. Martin screamed, "O my God!" and the daughter fainted and fell to the floor. Schultz sat up and was about to jump off the table when Dr. Friedson grabbed him around the legs and hugged him to his chest. When he looked down at the dog the large flap of skin had slipped to the side and was hanging in the air.

He stomped on the floor and called through the closed door, "Rachel, get in here; I need help!"

When Rachel walked in she couldn't believe her eyes. Mrs. Martin was pressed tight against the wall with her daughter lying on the floor between her legs. Dr. Friedson had the dog cradled in his arms with half of its skin hanging from its back; Dr. Friedson had a look on his face as if to say, "What just happened?"

Handing her the dog, he said, "Here, don't ask, just take Schultz and put him in a cage. He's hurt but he's not in shock and he is not dying."

He then walked around the table to tend to the girl just as she opened her eyes and tried to sit up. He told her to stay down for awhile and knelt over her as he folded a blanket and gently slid it under her head. Dr. Friedson noticed Mrs. Martin was a little pale and unsteady on her feet as she moved away from the wall and took a chair by the window.

When the situation had returned to a reasonable state of calm and the three of them had settled into comfortable chairs in Dr.

Friedson's office, Mrs. Martin tried to explain how Schultz had been injured. They assumed that Schultz decided to walk across the road just about the time a fast-moving car was approaching the store. The driver didn't see the dog in time and ran over him. Even though Schultz hunkered down, one of the cross members under the car must have caught him just behind the ears and peeled the skin of his back all the way to the base of the tail.

No one in the store heard a thud or cry or squeal and didn't realize the accident had happened until the driver let out a yell when she got out of the car and saw the dog trotting towards the house. As Mrs. Martin called the hospital, a customer and the car driver cared for Schultz and his injury. They replaced the flap of skin and tightly wrapped a towel around him to hold the flap in place. One of the daughters wrapped him in a blanket and sat with him on her lap on the way into town. Neither the mother nor the daughter had seen the entire loose flap of skin prior to the unwrapping at the hospital.

The surgery was quite simple, though tedious and stressful because there was some doubt if the procedure would be successful. The suturing would be similar to that used when grafting a piece of skin. The main concern was to try to establish an adequate blood supply to the flap of skin as quickly as possible to prevent it from drying up, dying, and sloughing away, so the sutures had to be placed close together to attach the skin to the vascular structures of the fat and muscles of the back.

Dr. Friedson started at the rear of the flap, near the base of the tail, and worked his way forward placing six sutures to a row across the back with each row being 1.5 inches apart. He ended up with eleven rows for a total of 44 sutures. He then used a total of 72 interlocking stitches to suture the edges of the skin together. Schultz was on the surgery table for a little over two hours, and

Dr. Friedson's fingers were noticeably tired when the procedure was completed.

Experience told Alton that pressure would have to be applied to the back to prevent the formation of air and fluid pockets. If this happened, the skin would separate from the subcutaneous tissues and the capillaries would not connect. Using an Ace bandage, he started at the base of the neck and wrapped it snuggly all the way back to the dog's hips, being careful not to cover the sheath and penis so Schultz could urinate freely. Strips of adhesive tape were placed from front to rear along the Ace bandage to keep it from separating.

Schultz was given 2ccs of penicillin, then put in a recovery cage where he would remain quiet for the next 48 hours. At this time, Schultz was given a good prognosis and Mrs. Martin was instructed to keep the dog inactive and quiet when she got him home returning in three days to have the bandage changed and the surgery evaluated.

Dr. Friedson considered this case to be one of the most unusual ones he had seen in his short career. He would feel extremely good about himself if the surgery was successful and Schultz had a complete recovery. The Martin family would be happy and appreciative and Schultz would go on to spend many more years dozing on the road in the sunshine, totally unconcerned about the cars coming and going.

EIGHTEEN

Nora and Tina showed up for their appointment right on schedule and appeared to be a little disappointed when Rachel told them that Dr. Branberg was gone for a week. The sisters had just returned from a vacation in Mazatlan, Mexico and wanted the doctor to do a physical and health check on two adorable dogs they had bought in Mexico and brought home with them.

The sisters, who never married, have lived together for the past twenty years. They always managed to have one or two pets of one kind or another, and the Valley Veterinary Hospital had been caring for their pets since they moved to town.

The ladies loved to travel, and it wasn't unusual for them to pick up a stray dog and bring it home. On one trip to Hawaii they had found a skinny dog running loose on a beach, and after much veterinary services and government paperwork they flew it home with them. When they got to the USA it had to be quarantined for four months.

Rachel opened the office door and announced to Dr. Friedson that the sisters were in the exam room. They had a small carrier, which supposedly housed two little dogs.

Alton walked into the small room, smiled, extended his hand to both sisters and asked if they were having a pleasant day. He knew they would rather have Dr. Branberg, so he was always kind and flattering, hoping to win them over.

"We just got back from Mazatlan," Nora piped up, "and

outwitted the customs in Tijuana by smuggling two Chihuahuas home with us." She giggled as she put her hand to her mouth.

"We didn't really smuggle them, Nora. They didn't ask, and we didn't tell them," Tina explained.

"Just a minute," Dr. Friedson interrupted. "Let's start from the beginning. It will be easier for me if I get a little history and know how and where you got these dogs."

Nora always was the more outspoken of the two, so she started. "One afternoon we decided to take a drive out into the country and we came upon a small roadside cafe and stopped to have a cool drink."

"It was just a soda, Nora, don't make it sound like we were drinking alcohol and driving," said Tina.

"While we were sitting at the table, a young man came in carrying a box and kneeled by our table."

Tina added, "He surprised us because he spoke very good English."

"He said he had two dogs he had to find a place for and he would sell them to us for only a few dollars if we would take them and give them a good home. He said they were very well bred and came from a long line of show dogs. When we asked them what breed they were, he said they were Chihuahuas."

Tina corrected her again. "Actually, he said they were Toy Mexican Hairless Chihuahuas."

"Anyway, he said he would give us a bargain at what amounted to $10.00 a piece in American money, which included enough food and treats until we got home. He showed them to us and let us hold them, and we didn't have the heart to turn him down."

"They were so ugly they were cute," Tina said with a short laugh.

"How did you get them across the border?" Dr. Friedson asked.

"We put them in a box and hid them under our luggage," Nora said.

Tina shrugged her shoulders, "The customs agent didn't ask if we had pets and they didn't look in the trunk. We were crossing our fingers that the dogs wouldn't bark."

"Well, let's take a look at these two illegal aliens," Dr. Friedson joked.

Nora put the box on the floor, opened the lid, scooped up the two animals in both hands and placed them on the table. Tina opened her mouth to speak, but she was taken aback by Dr. Friedson's surprised and almost scared expression. He slapped his hand to his forehead and in a shout that frightened them both said, "Get out of here now. Hurry, leave the room. Leave those things right there. Do as I say!"

He half shoved and pushed them as he followed them out the door.

"What are you doing?" Nora protested. "Those are our dogs!"

"Those are not dogs, Nora, they are domestic Mexican rats. They run wild in the Mexican desert and are semi-dangerous. They can carry all kinds of diseases; some we don't even know how to treat."

"Oh, my God!" Tina shouted and ran into the waiting room holding her mouth as if she was going to be sick.

"But he said they were Chihuahua dogs. And they are kind and cuddly," Nora said, looking confused.

"Nora, come and sit down. There is no hairless Chihuahua breed. They are short hair or long hair, none with very little hair like those rats. Chihuahuas have short fluffy tails, big round eyes and large bat-like ears. Their legs are long and their feet are big with long toes. I can show you a picture. Those are rats. They have long skinny tails, short small ears, short legs and beady eyes."

"But why aren't they wild? They didn't try to bite or run away. They sat on our lap and liked to be petted and scratched."

"Don't try to justify our actions, Nora," Tina said as she began to sob. "They're rats. And to think I held them, I fed them, and loved them. It's disgusting. I feel dirty and sick all over." She put her head in her hands and sobbed even harder. Rachel came around the corner and put her arm around Tina's shoulder. "Let's go into the office, Tina. I have some tissues and you can wash up."

"What do we do now, Dr. Fried? Do you think we have been exposed to anything? Are there tests we should take?" Nora asked. She seemed genuinely concerned.

"Let's go into the office and we'll talk about it with Tina."

Dr. Friedson explained, "There are semi-domestic rats, like those, that live in and hang around the farm buildings in the rural areas in western Mexico. Kids catch them, tame them, play with them and, as you have experienced, sell them to naïve tourists. Fortunately, those that are raised by these kids are usually harmless and are no threat health-wise."

"So do you think we are okay?" Tina asked.

"I think so. I suggest you go home and take a long hot shower with lots of strong soap. Check yourself carefully each day for any pimples or rash, and call your doctor if you see or feel anything unusual. Disinfect with Clorox any area where those guys have slept or gone potty. Throw away their bedding and feeding dishes. Just to be sure; don't be too careful."

"What will you do with them?" Nora asked in a quiet voice. It sounded like she hoped they wouldn't have to be put to sleep.

"I will examine them for parasites such as lice and ticks; if they have any, I will let you know. Then I will euthanize them and cremate the bodies." Alton didn't want to worry them so he spoke matter-of-factly as if this was something he did every day.

Rachel had served each of them a cup of coffee, and soon the sisters had collected themselves and accepted the fact that they had been taken by a con man. They were relieved to know that probably no damage had been done except for the loss of a few dollars and an insult to their intelligence.

They had no desire to say goodbye to their would-be pets and left saying they had learned a valuable lesson. They assured Dr. Friedson and Rachel that they would not be bringing home any more strays from other countries.

NINETEEN

After the sisters left, Alton and Rachel talked about how bizarre was what they had just seen and heard.. How two mature, intelligent people, who have been around dogs most of their life, could fall for such a scam. They were fortunate that no one got injured and that they didn't lose more money than they did.

As Alton stood behind the reception counter, he glanced up and the POP rack caught his eye. He saw Donna Hoople's card filed on end. "Rachel, have you talked to the Hooples recently?" he asked.

"No, they haven't called since you were out there. I assumed you had been in contact with them."

Alton reached up, took the card and dialed the number.

"Hello," answered a familiar voice.

"Hi, Donna, this is Dr. Fried. I'm calling to inquire about our patient."

"Oh, hi! Well, I think the news is good. Everything is going just about the way you said it would. We keep her standing in her stall and she moves around by pivoting on her front legs. She can move them backwards a little but I haven't seen any big movements forward."

"How are the wounds doing? Is there any sign of weeping or infection?" He was hoping she would say no.

"I don't think so. We are continuing to put the aloe vera gel on twice a day and keep it wrapped. Oh, that is one question we had. Do you think we have to keep it bandaged? She doesn't lie down so it can't get dirty."

"Are the tissues quite dry? When you put on the gel does it stick or run down the legs?" he asked.

"Oh, yes. We really pack it in and it stays there. Of course, when it gets warm it runs a little, but most of it stays. We are using a lot of bandage material and it would be nice if we could get by without it."

"Well, why don't you try it? I'll get up there in the next few days and evaluate the progress. Does she seem to be comfortable and happy?"

"She would like to be out with her buddies. She whinnies for them so I am sure she is a little lonely, but otherwise I would say she is content. Thanks for calling, Dr. Fried. Make it up if you can."

When Alton put the card back in the slot, he noticed the card for Mrs. Martin. He took it out and saw a progress report attached. "I see Mrs. Martin called," he said, showing the card to Rachel.

"Yeh, that was yesterday."

He read the note half out loud and half to himself. Schultz was running around as if nothing had happened. The stitches were holding and looking good, and there was no sign of weeping. The only concern was a spot just back of the head where the skin was turning black and seemed to be dry and hard. She speculated that that was the spot where the car cross-member first struck, and the skin was badly bruised and would probably die. Unless something changed there was no cause for concern. She would be in the first of the week to have the stitches removed and have him checked over.

The POP (phone on progress) was a slotted, wooden rack that hung on the wall near the door behind Rachel's reception desk. The personal records of patients that had been in recently for surgery or treatment were placed there for easy access for follow-up phone calls. Two or three days after the patient had gone home from having work done, Rachel or one of the doctors would call the owner for a progress report. The policy served several purposes. It made the owner feel good knowing that the doctor was concerned and took the time to inquire about their pet. The call gave the doctor an opportunity to pick up on any problems that may be developing and nip them in the bud. It gave the owner an opportunity to ask questions about concerns or problems they were experiencing involving procedures that were performed. When the doctor felt the animal was well on the road to recovery, the card was removed and put in the client record cabinet.

The wooden rack was purposely placed in a very conspicuous place near the phone, so the cards would not be forgotten and there would be no excuses not to call the client. The way the hospital was laid out meant that everyone moving about the hospital would pass by and could not help but notice the cards in the rack.

The patient waiting room and the reception desk were in the middle of the building with the front door facing the street where the clients parked. The east side of the building consisted of the doctor's offices and the night attendant's apartment which was made up of a kitchen, bedroom, and a bathroom. There was another bathroom in the middle of the building right next to the reception desk. Behind the desk was a door leading into the laboratory and a small work area. An outside door opened to a small storage shed and parking area where the doctors parked their vehicles.

A hall going west from the reception area had a door on the right opening into the exam room, and two doors on the left opening into two dog boarding pens. At the end of the hall was a door leading into the hospital work area and surgery prep. Two doors on the right opened into the surgery room and the equipment and pharmacy supply room. A door on the south wall led to a larger room housing the large autoclave, the X-ray machine and a grooming table. In the corner was a small X-ray film developing room. In back of this were the kennel area, the exercise runs and a bathing area with a tub and dryers.

The hospital consisted of a total of 1700 square feet sitting on approximately one-half acre of city property on the south side of the main road going west out of town. It was a good location because the main highway ran in front of the building, making it convenient to get to and enabling the doctors to get out of town quickly and easily when making farm calls.

Because of the floor plan of the hospital and the medical preferences of the doctors, the traffic flow throughout the hospital was not a problem. No one kept running into one another. Dr. Friedson was comfortable doing the treatments and surgery so most of his time was spent in the working areas of the hospital. Dr. Branberg loved the diagnostic and laboratory part of the practice so he did most of the examinations and testing in the rooms off to the side, and Rachel spent most of her day in the waiting and reception area. It was a workable situation for everyone concerned. Dr. Friedson often thought of what might happen if the practice got so busy they had to hire a third veterinarian. Would everything be so neat and tidy? He had heard many stories of multiple doctor clinics where things didn't go well because of accusations, jealousies, personality conflicts and all sorts of problems. He was relieved knowing that, so far, the two doctors could handle the workload, although there were recognizable signs that things could change.

TWENTY

As Dr. Friedson drove home on Highway 9 along the north end of the lake, he thought about how difficult it was, especially for the elderly, to make drastic changes. Changing something that has been part of their life for many years is not an easy decision to make. For the next several days Edna would be watching her goats with a critical eye and evaluating the results of the new procedures, trying to decide if the new was more successful than the old.

Alton thought back to some of the decisions he had had to make concerning veterinary medicine during the eight years since he left school. The more he thought about it, the more he realized there were not that many major changes. The first one that came to mind was switching to disposable hypodermic needles. Dr. Branberg was reluctant to make the change because of the cost. Each needle packaged in a plastic sterile container carried a price tag of eighteen cents, which he figured could cost the hospital a minimum of $60.00 a month - more than he was willing to spend. Alton argued that sharpening needles over and over again and sterilizing them in the autoclave was a waste of time and not always that effective. Some of the larger gauge needles never got real sharp, and sterility was always a major question. At slack times during the day, one of the doctors would sharpen and sterilize old needles. This involved rubbing the tip on a wet stone until the point was sharp, then putting them in a metal box, placing them in the Castle autoclave and cooking them at the required time and pressure to insure sterilization. The whole procedure could take thirty minutes or more and was not one that either doctor enjoyed doing. After Dr. Branberg was convinced to make the change, he admitted that it should have been done much, much earlier.

Dr. Branberg had dragged his feet again when Alton suggested they switch to disposable plastic syringes. When Alton joined the hospital, injections were given with glass, nylon or metal syringes. Just as with the needles, these had to be cleaned and sterilized after every use. It was not only time-consuming but after a period of time the syringes became difficult to use. After several autoclavings, the nylon syringes became sticky and the plungers were hard to push. The rubber washers in the metal syringes would swell and cause problems. The barrels of the glass syringes would become weak and crack during sterilization. When Alton began hinting that disposable syringes would be much more efficient and time saving, Dr. Branberg would just let on that he wasn't listening. When Alton suggested that they make the change, Dr. Branberg complained about the price. He stated that glass syringes had been used for years and if they were good enough then, they were good enough now. But it was mostly because of the expense that Dr. Branberg held his ground, until Alton convinced him that the plastic syringes could be autoclaved over and over again. Although the manufacturers and distributors sold them as disposable plastic syringes, they were of such high quality that they could be reused. A bag of 100 would last a long time. Finally, after much discussion Dr. Branberg gave in and after a couple of weeks of enjoying the ease and efficiency of the new syringes, he confessed it was a worthwhile luxury and the change was long overdue.

If Alton thought convincing Dr. Branberg to switch to disposable products was difficult, he had a real battle coming up when proposing some of the newer general anesthetics. When

Alton hired on at the Valley Veterinary Hospital, he thought he had stepped back into the dark ages when he found out the anesthetic used for small animal surgery was ether. He once whispered to Rachel he was surprised it wasn't chloroform. In school he had been taught how to use the inhalant gas machines and the doses and precautions of the several injectable anesthetics. Ether was considered obsolete, and most veterinarians and hospitals refused to use it because it is highly inflammable even to the point of being explosive. Many animals died on the surgery table because their respiration under ether anesthetic wasn't monitored properly and they went into cardiac arrest. Although it had been used effectively for many years, it was not a safe product.

At the Valley Veterinary Hospital the anesthetic procedure was quite simple, although at times it did involve a little struggle. In a drawer in the presurgery room were four canvas bags: one small enough to tightly fit over the nose of a small cat, one to fit over the nose of a large cat or small dog, and two for medium and large dogs. A wad of cotton was stuffed into the closed end of the bag, and both were soaked with ether when ready for use.

A cat being readied for surgery would be zippered into a canvas bag and held tightly while the nose bag and cotton soaked with ether was placed over its nose. After an initial short struggle, the cat would relax and go to sleep. If the cat began to wake up during surgery, the bag was put over its nose again for a short period of time. The recovery period was quite short and occurred without much of a struggle. All in all the procedure was effective, inexpensive and safe, as long as everyone involved was cautious.

One afternoon Dr. Friedson was spaying a cat when Dr. Branberg walked into the surgery just to chat. He had just returned from lunch with a friend who treated him to a good cigar. He stood puffing on the cigar and when he reached to take it from his mouth, some hot ashes fell off and landed on the ether bag, which was pushed over the cat's nose and face. Suddenly there was a loud poof, a cloud of smoke and the bag burst into flames. Dr. Branberg quickly pulled the bag from the cat and threw it on the floor and stomped out the fire with his boot. Dr. Friedson jumped back, dropping the carmalt forceps and shielding his face with a gloved hand. No serious harm was done, but the flames did burn the cat's whiskers and singe the hair on its face.

The one good thing that came out of the incident was the realization how dangerous ether could be. After apologizing for being so careless, Dr. Branberg admitted that it was probably time to change to a safer anesthetic. A product called Surital arrived at the hospital a short time later and was used extensively for many years.

It was because of Surital that Dr. Branberg agreed to purchase an inhalation gas anesthetic machine. Surital was a great general anesthetic, but it had one downfall - it had to be given intravenously. If a small amount was injected into the interstitial tissues surrounding the vein, it could cause a serious reaction with swelling, redness, pain and sloughing of the skin. This made for a real challenge when trying to hit the radial vein on a small cat. The patient had to be held perfectly still while the doctor inserted a 22-gauge needle into the threadlike vein and slowly injected the correct dosage for the weight of the cat. With some practice it was accomplished without a hitch, but Dr. Branberg didn't do much small animal surgery and when he had to, he got quite nervous thinking about the anesthetic. After a few minor mishaps and some prodding from Dr. Friedson, he agreed to purchase a machine. A sales representative was able to locate a used Halothane machine and the hospital purchased it for $700.00. Dr. Branberg considered it one of the better purchases he had made in some time.

The one time Dr. Friedson and Dr. Branberg had a heated

disagreement happened one Saturday afternoon involved a drastic change in hospital policy, and Dr. Branberg had a hard time accepting it.

Dr. Friedson was called out to Ron Vanpol's dairy to treat a large, heavy-milking Holstein for milk fever. The cow was down in the loafing shed and Mr. Vanpol wasn't busy at the time, so the he and Dr. Friedson walked together to the shed to treat the cow and have some time to visit. As they talked, Alton went through the treatment routine, one he could do with his eyes shut, and as he did so he noticed that Ron was paying very close attention to what he was doing, and asking some very specific questions.

Alton used a set of nose tongs to tie the cows head to its rear leg, disinfected the jugular groove with alcohol, put pressure on the lower part of the vein to enlarge it, and then watched to make sure he had a good flow of blood as he inserted the catheter into the vein.

"Is that a special needle you use to stick into the vein?" Ron asked as he bent down to examine it.

"It's a needle with a plastic tube running through it. It's called a catheter and is designed to run further into the vein to prevent leakage," Alton replied. "It isn't absolutely necessary. Most times I use just the needle, but if the cow is restless or wants to jump up, then the catheter is nice to have inserted." Alton pulled the rubber stopper from the 500cc bottle of calcium gluconate, attached it to the IV set and inserted the free end into the needle protruding from the jugular vein. Holding the bottle above the cow's head, he knelt on the ground and took out his stethoscope.

"I understand that the calcium has to go into the vein, is that correct?" Ron stood by the cow's head watching the bubbles rising in the coffee-colored liquid in the bottle.

"Oh, yeah, for it to be effective that is the way it has to be administered. See, it says right here on the label," Alton pointed to the warning along the bottom of the paper. "For veterinary use only. For intravenous injection."

"I know it's calcium that you have to inject that makes the cow better, but exactly what is it?" Ron asked inquisitively.

"It's a mixture of several things, but you are right, it is the calcium the cow needs to get back on her feet. Here, you can read the label. We buy it by the case from the Fort Dodge representative."

"Would it be possible for me to buy it?" Ron asked.

Alton looked at him for a long time with a quizzical look on his face, and then asked, "Why would you want to buy it?"

"Well, to be honest with you, I am thinking about treating my own milk fevers. I have been giving it some thought for some time now and watching you and asking questions. I see no reason why I can't do it."

Alton didn't know what to say, so he put the stethoscope in his ears and began listening to the cow's heart. He faintly heard Ron going on.

"I know the Tellison brothers treat their own cows. They told me they buy the calcium from the Co-op Farm Supply. If you would just give me a few tips and warn me of things not to do, I think I could manage."

Alton laid the stethoscope down and without looking up said, "Ron you are a competent, capable dairyman. You have a degree in animal husbandry, for Pete's sake. I know you can treat these milk fevers just as well as I can. And sure, I'll teach you how to do it and tell you all about it, but there is one problem."
"What's that?" Ron asked.

"Dr. Branberg is not going to be very happy about it, and when he finds out I am the one who encouraged you to do this, he will be all over me."

"He has to know that this sort of thing is coming. Farmers

and dairymen aren't what they used to be. Kids are coming out of school with degrees in agriculture and animal science, and they aren't dummies. They know and can learn how to do things our parents and grandparents never thought of doing. How difficult is it to put a needle in a cow's vein and run in 500cc's of calcium?" Ron questioned

"I agree with you one hundred percent, but when Dr. Branberg hears about it or asks me about it, he will be pretty upset when I tell him," responded Dr. Friedson.

Dr. Friedson accepted the fact that more and more dairymen were doing their own treatments, and mostly out of necessity. The price of milk hadn't risen substantially in years and their expenses kept going up and up. In order to stay in business they had to cut corners and lower their overhead, and doing some of their own veterinary work was one way to accomplish this. Many dairymen were treating milk fevers, and mastitis, trimming feet, delivering calves, dehorning heifers, castrating bull calves, relieving bloat, and opening abscesses, and some were even doing their own inseminating. It was changing with the times.

Back at the hospital Alton poured himself a cup of coffee, walked into the lab and sat against the edge of the desk. Dr. Branberg was at his microscope reading milk sample slides and chewing on a toothpick, which he often did when concentrating on a project.

"Ron Vanpol told me today he is going to start treating his own milk fevers," Alton said as he picked up a veterinary journal and pretended to study the picture on the cover.

"He won't know how unless somebody shows him. Then he will have trouble with the first one and he'll be sorry," Rand replied.

"I know several farms that do much of their own work, and they seem to do alright."

"You might think so, but they make lots of mistakes. It's just that you never hear about it because they aren't going to talk about it or admit it."

"Well, Ron was asking me a lot of questions today about what kind of calcium to give and how to give it and asked me outright if I thought he was capable of doing it," said Alton.

"I hope you weren't helpful and discouraged him from trying it."

"No, I showed him what I was using, told him it wasn't brain surgery and said he shouldn't have any problems."

Dr. Branberg stopped chewing on the toothpick, sat motionless for a while, then slowly pushed his chair back and turned towards Alton. He had a disgusted look on his face and spoke in a slow quiet voice.

"I'm really disappointed. I have spent years building this practice and giving excellent service to the farmers, and I refuse to sit by and have it taken away from me. If we encourage the dairymen to do their own treatments and teach them how to do it, do you realize how much money we would lose in a month? It could set me back a significant amount."

"With me, Rand, it is not so much the money as the time. Do you enjoy crawling out of bed at five in the morning, or being called out Sunday afternoon, or in the middle of a nice dinner party? And the big percentage of those calls is milk fevers. Think about it. We charge a total of $13.00 to treat a milk fever. Five dollars of that are expenses, so we profit $8.00. Wouldn't you rather give up the $8.00 than leave a party, run home and change, walk out into a muddy field in the dark with a flashlight to find a cow down at the far end of the pasture, and get soaked and cold while sitting in the rain running in the calcium? I know I would. Besides I have a suggestion as to how we can make up for it."

"I know what you are saying," Dr. Branberg replied, "but

there is the satisfaction and the pride involved knowing that you saved a cow's life and you gave that dairyman excellent service when he needed it."

Alton refilled his coffee cup, returned and said, "Do you know what most of those dairymen are thinking when you drive away? I bet they aren't thinking about the great service you gave but how the trip cost them $13.00 and they could have done the job themselves for practically nothing."

"What's this suggestion you have?" Dr. Branberg asked.

Alton walked around the desk and stood in front of Dr. Branberg, stretched out his arms and asked, "What is the one thing that keeps dairymen in business?"

"Producing milk. Selling milk," Dr. Branberg replied.

"Yes, but what is it that makes it possible for them to produce milk?" Alton pressed for a right answer.

"They have cows that give milk, and hopefully they are good cows that give thousands of pounds a year," Dr. Branberg was getting a little irritated from the quizzing.

"And what would be the one main reason why a cow would not give milk?" Alton had a smile on his face because he knew that Rand was finally catching on to what he was getting at.

"If they don't get pregnant and don't freshen, they won't come into their milk and eventually the dairyman would be out of business. So how does that help compensate for the financial loss from losing the milk fever cases?" Dr. Branberg asked with a little more interest in what Alton was suggesting.

"We become fertility specialists. I would venture to say that you know more about infertility and how to get a cow pregnant better than any other vet in the county. This is one area that the dairymen will never master. They will not learn to pregnancy-check a cow, they do not have the schooling or practice to diagnose ovarian or uterine problems, and they do not have the anatomical or pharmacological knowledge to treat an infertility problem. They need veterinarians to get their infertile cows pregnant and keep them pregnant so their cows will calf, come into their milk, and be a producer."

"So just exactly what is it that you are proposing?" Dr. Branberg asked.

"It is pertinent that the owner knows whether or not a cow is pregnant. It's his livelihood. We offer that service and charge $2.00 for a rectal pregnancy exam. If she isn't pregnant, we find out why and treat her so she will conceive. For this we charge from $3.00 to $5.00. We get a gross amount of $8.00 for what it took us four years and many dollars to learn and for which no one but us knows how to do. For this specialty service I think we should receive more than we get for treating a milk fever. Therefore, let's substantially raise the price of our pregnancy checks and infertility work. It wouldn't have to be much to cover the loss from the eclampsia cases."

"You know, I think I like it. Not that I approve of teaching the cattlemen how to treat their own milk fevers, but I think your proposal has some merit," Dr. Branberg leaned back in his chair and stuck a pencil in his mouth.

"To start with, we should make an effort to educate ourselves and polish our skills to become highly efficient in diagnosing and treating infertility and making sure the farmers are familiar with what we know and can do. I think they would be receptive to changes when they know they are getting the best service available." Alton was getting more enthused the longer he talked.

"Well, let's think about it and put some ideas down on paper." Dr. Branberg bent over the microscope as if to discontinue the conversation.

Alton wanted the last word. "Rand, with your experience

and knowledge of pathology and my practical skills we could be an unbeatable team. I firmly believe that in ten to fifteen years, infertility in Holstein cows is going to be the veterinarian's bread and butter."

TWENTY ONE

I t was 11:00 in the morning. Dr. Branberg was out at a dairy collecting milk samples, and Alton and Rachel had just put Schultz on the table for a check-up when the bell on the front door tinkled. Rachel stepped out into the hall to see a Visula being pulled through the door by a stout lady who turned and shouted, "Put this stupid dog to sleep. I never want to see it again!" She dropped the leash on the floor and slammed the door behind her.

Rachel hurried to the front window to see Mrs. Maglie get into her car and drive away. She was sure it was Laura Maglie but she wasn't driving her familiar 1957 green two-door Chev; it looked like a new car.

She turned to see Rosie; at least she looked like Rosie, sitting in the middle of the waiting room with a sorrowful look and shaking as if she had been very bad and was being severely punished.

"Boy that was strange!" Rachel announced as she led the Visula into the prep room.

"What happened? I heard some shouting."

"I'm sure it was Mrs. Maglie. She more or less threw this dog into the waiting room and said put it to sleep. She didn't ever want to see it again. I'm sure this is her dog Rosie."

"Let me see. Here, take Schultz." He knelt down to look closely at the dog because practically all Visulas look alike from a distance. Yes, she had been spayed, he thought to himself as he ran his fingers over the stainless steel sutures lying just under the skin. It could be from his surgery but some other clinics also closed the peritoneum with steel sutures, although it wasn't common. Most doctors used cat gut. Then he remembered a procedure he had done on Rosie about a year ago. He opened her mouth and, to his relief, saw a large gap with no teeth on the right upper jaw.

He looked up at Rachel and said, "Would you please get me Laura's records. Didn't we pull some teeth on Rosie about a year ago?"

Rachel opened the folder and sure enough Alton had extracted the pr-molar and the large masticating molar on the right maxillary jaw fifteen months earlier. Further proof was that she had a large scar on her lower right rear leg where a skin tumor had been removed.

"Are we going to put her to sleep?" Rachel asked in a somber voice.

Alton was in a teasing mood and with a serious, professional look on his face said, "The client is always right and, regardless of how we think or feel, we must respect their wishes."

"But Rosie is just a young dog. Laura loves her like her own children. She isn't sick, she isn't lame, and there is nothing wrong with her. She couldn't have done something so terrible to die for it," Rachel was pleading.

"I don't know the circumstances, Rachel, but if she says put the dog down then we have no alternative but to put the dog down," being more stern than usual.

Rachel was still pleading, "If she had seriously bitten someone I could understand, but Rosie is the most gentle and loving creature you could ever meet. She wouldn't hurt anyone or anything. Would you, Rosie?" she bent down and patted the dog's head and gave her a kiss on the nose. When Alton saw tears welling up in her eyes his voice softened, he put his hand on Rosie's head and said, "No, we are not going to put her to sleep. Whatever she did will soon be forgiven and Mrs. Maglie will be on the phone in a couple of hours. For the life of me I can't think of what the dog could have done to upset her so. She has had Rosie for ten years and has put up with all her bad habits."

"I noticed she was driving a new car," Rachel added as if to offer a hint of an explanation.

"That could be it. Rosie may have left a 'deposit' on the back seat in protest to the new vehicle. Animals do that sometimes when they are upset with a change in their life. You know, like male cats will spray around the house when there is a major change in their environment. When you think about it, the only car Rosie knows is that green Chev. That was the only car the Maglies had when they got her as a puppy and she went everywhere in that car. It was like a second home to her."

"Well, when Laura calls to give her a stay of execution we will get the facts. But what if she doesn't call? Then what?" she asked, obviously concerned. Just then the phone rang. "That's her. It'll be all right, Rosie. She will have calmed down by now and she is on her way to pick you up." But the call wasn't Mrs. Maglie and Rosie's future was still up in the air.

Alton finished examining Schultz and was pleased that he was recovering as well as expected. As he finished caring for the other in-house patients, morning turned to noon, noon turned to afternoon, soon it was closing time and yet no word from the Maglie household. Alton walked back to the kennel area, and being as sympathetic and reassuring as possible, he let Rosie out for a run, gave her fresh water and a bowl of Purina Dog Chow and said goodnight.

The next morning Rachel had barely unlocked the front door when Laura Maglie nonchalantly strolled in, walked up to the counter and calmly said, "I know you didn't put my Rosie to sleep; you know me too well. So I will just pay the bill and take her home." Offering no explanation, she just stood quietly thumbing through her purse as if looking for her check-book.

Rachel stood dumbfounded. She desperately wanted an explanation but didn't know what to say. Laura didn't offer any, and her aloof presence was as if nothing happened and she was just here to pick up her dog after a night's stay. After a short silence Rachel said, "I don't know the charge. I will have to get Dr. Friedson."

When Alton heard that she had come for her dog, he hurried to the waiting room and without a greeting or a "How are you?" he happily said, "No, we didn't put Rosie to sleep. We knew there was a logical explanation and you would be back to pick her up. But what a mystery! None of us could think of a thing Rosie could possibly do to cause such a drastic reaction on your part. So we made her comfortable and assured her that you would be back."

Mrs. Maglie leaned against the counter, hung her head and said, "I am terribly embarrassed and ashamed about the way I acted. I was so upset and so angry I just lost my head and acted without thinking."

"Well, what happened?" Alton asked.

"It's that new car. She doesn't like it and she showed it yesterday morning." Alton and Rachel glanced at each other as if to say, "Yeah, we guessed it had something to do with the car."

"As you know, the only car we have had since we got Rosie was that green Chevy, and she thought of it as her second home. She practically lived in it and I can understand why she would be upset if it was taken from her. But to do what she did is inexcusable." She walked to the window and stood looking outside. "I had to go to Safeway so I put her in the car, as I have done for years, and left her there while I shopped for the groceries. When I came out, she had completely destroyed the inside of the car. She had bitten chunks out of the leather dash, ripped the cloth off the roof, chewed the leather off the steering wheel, torn the cloth off the seats, and completely destroyed two arm rests. This was my new car. I had had it only three days."

Rachel walked over and put her arm around Laura's shoulder. "You had a right to be angry and it is understandable you would react the way you did."

Pointing out the window she said, "This is the first new car we have ever had." She lowered herself into one of the chairs and hid her face in her hands as she started to cry. "Then I did the most unforgivable thing- I hit her. I slapped her several times on her head and said she was a terrible, nasty dog. How could I hit her? She's my baby." While she sat sobbing with Rachel trying to comfort her, Alton went and brought Rosie to the waiting room. She immediately ran over to her mistress, snuggled her nose into her hands and laid her head on her lap.

What a reunion! The room was filled with sobbing, laughing, shouting and yapping as the four of them hugged and danced to celebrate the joyous occasion.

There was nothing more to say or do. Mrs. Maglie took Rosie to the car and lovingly put her in the tattered front seat and slowly drove away.

TWENTY TWO

Early morning was Alton's favorite time of the day. On work days he would often have a quick breakfast then drive to the hospital hoping to get caught up on some laboratories and paper work before jumping into the hustle and bustle of another busy day. He could usually bank on two hours of peace and quiet but even though the sign on the door said "open at 8:00 am" there were always a few who began banging on the door long before, thinking they were special and had certain privileges. Clients with emergencies were excused but why wouldn't they call first?

It was shortly before 8:00 and Alton was in the laboratory reading mastitis slides when he heard some scuffling at the front door. There was some grunting, banging against the door and rattling of the door knob. Alton looked around the corner and through the window on the front door he saw a large man trying to open the door while struggling not to drop a large dog that was slipping out of his arms.

"Hello," Alton said.

At first the man didn't speak, just looked around the room then gently laid the dog on the floor.

"Is there a vet here?" He asked after catching his breath.

"Yes, I am the doctor." Alton replied. "You got a problem?"

"Yeah, my dog has multiple cuts and it could be bad. He needs some care."

Dr. Friedson didn't recognize the man, couldn't recall seeing him around and the dog didn't look familiar. It appeared to part terrier, like an Airedale mixed with a long haired breed, perhaps a Shepherd.

"You haven't been in before? Or have you?"

"No, do you have a problem with that?" he blurted.

Just then Rachel stepped into the waiting room, "Hi, got a sick dog? O my goodness he looks injured. Got a sore foot? She was her usual cheerful self.

"He got drug behind a truck and I need a vet to look at him. He has lost some blood."

When Alton heard the problem he leaned over the counter and took a closer look at the dog. His back legs were covered with blood and his face was badly swollen. He listened as Rachel filled out the client card.

Evidently the man, Mr. Gill Gore, and a friend had planned a trip to Anacortes for an afternoon of fishing, and decided to take the dog along. They had tied the dog in the back of the pickup next to the cab and told him to lie down. Somewhere, somehow he either chewed through or broke one of the ropes and either fell or jumped out of the truck. Neither one of the men knew how long the dog had been dragged behind the truck.

At one point a car pulled alongside with its horn honking and the man in its passenger seat pointing frantically to the back of the pickup. He rolled down his window and hollered,

"Your dog, your dog!"

The men pulled over to the side of the road and stopped. The dog was lying partly in the ditch beside the hind wheel of the truck. The rope had pulled the collar tight around his neck, his head was swollen and he was gasping for air. His rear legs were bloody, his fur was full of weeds, grass, gravel, and small sticks. His eyes were swollen shut and he had a long open cut on his right ear. At first the men thought the dog was dead but seeing him breathing, they realized he was alive. They packed him into the truck and hurried to the hospital.

Rachel took his name, address, telephone number and the information about the dog. He was a six-year-old Airedale mix named Rio and Mr. Gore had owned him since he was a six week old puppy. Rachel thought Mr. Gore may have been in a mild state of shock because he was a little hesitant when giving his address and phone number. She didn't dwell on it as it certainly would be understandable considering what he had just been through.

Alton helped Mr. Gore carry Rio into the surgery prep room and lay him on the table. As Alton began examining Rio's injuries, Mr. Gore leaned back against the sink counter, folded his arms across his chest and began talking.

"You know doc, I wouldn't do anything to hurt Rio. He's been my pal since he was a baby. He goes everywhere with me. I considered leaving him home today because he doesn't much like the boat, but when I was ready to go he looked at me with those big eyes and I just couldn't leave him behind."

"Could you not see in your mirror that you were dragging him in the ditch?" Dr. Friedson asked as he picked up a rear foot.

"No. Jim and I were talking and I wasn't paying attention. Doc you have to do everything possible to fix him up; no matter what it takes." He reached over and laid a hand on the dog's head, "He's my buddy, aren't you big guy?"

"He's pretty scraped up but none of the injuries are life threatening and there doesn't appear to be any fractures. There's going to be a lot of cleaning, debriding and suturing."

Mr. Gore stepped from the counter and confronted Dr. Friedson face to face, "Doc, whatever it takes and whatever it costs I don't care. Money is not a problem. Spend what you have to, he's worth every penny. Do you understand? Do what it takes." He put his hand on Alton's shoulder.

"Let me show you the injuries and explain what has to be done and give some estimate on healing time. First we will have to treat Rio for shock and give him a couple of hours rest before starting any procedures. His head is bruised and swollen and he has a broken right upper canine tooth. This cut on his ear will have to be sutured. A lot of hair and skin has been scraped off the chest but there are no broken ribs and no puncture wounds. These should heal quickly and the hair should grow back. The worst areas are the right hip and the rear feet; areas where the skin lies practically next to the bone with no muscle or fat for protection. As you can see the skin is completely gone, exposing the bones, ligaments, and tendons. On the right foot the toe nails are completely worn off and will not grow back, because the tips of the toes are gone. You see all this sand packed under and between the ligaments and foot bones? That will all have to be picked out by hand with tweezers. All the loose skin will have to be cut away and the feet will have to be wrapped with moisturizing ointments. Rio will be in surgery for a few hours; there will be fluids, antibiotics and bandages."

"Doc, as I said before, this guy is part of me. Money is not a problem. Just make him better."

"Okay, then I guess we better get started. We will keep him today and tomorrow and you can pick him up Wednesday afternoon. Call tomorrow or stop by if you wish. What it'll cost I don't."

Mr. Gore put up his hand, "Just give me the bill. No explanations necessary."

Rio was ready to go when Mr. Gore walked in at 2:30 Wednesday afternoon. He was stiff and sore and a little depressed but he perked up when he saw his master.

"Hey buddy how ya doin?" Mr. Gore knelt on the floor and

was careful not to pet the dog where it might hurt. "He looks great doc; I'll take good care of him."

"Rachel will give you the statement and the instructions for post surgical care. It's going to take a couple of months for those sores to heal."

"I'll do it and I'll let you know how he does." Mr. Gore stood up, "Give me the bill young lady, I'll take care of that then carry Rio out to the truck." He put his hand in his back pocket, then his two front pockets and patted his shirt pockets, "Oh no! My wallet. Just a minute." He walked to the window and motioned to the man in the truck. Jim walked in and with a questionable look said, "What?"

"Do you have my wallet? I can't find it."

"It was on the table. I thought you picked it up."

"Listen miss, Rachel isn't it? Seems I left my wallet and money at home. I'll take Rio to the house, make him comfortable then come right back with the cash. Give me the slip. Jim can you stay with Rio while I run back here and settle up?"

"Sure." Jim replied

"Is that okay with you?" He looked at Rachel. "Would the doc let me do that? I won't be more than 45 minutes."

"Sure. Just remember we close at 5:00."

They left with Jim driving and Mr. Gore holding Rio on his lap; making for a crowded front seat.

At 5:15 Alton walked up to the front desk and asked Rachel, "When Mr. Gore came back to settle his bill, did he pay all of it or just part?"

"He didn't come back," Rachel said reaching to lock the front door.

"I thought he was going to be back within the hour?"

"That's what he said but he hasn't shown."

A week went by and still no word or visit from Mr. Gil Gore.

"Hey Rachel, you better call our friend with the Airedale and find out how the patient is doing and when we can expect a payment."

"Funny you should ask. I called his number this morning and a lady with a pleasant, clear voice said, "I'm sorry, the number you are trying to reach is no longer in service." I checked the phone book and there was a Joe Gore but not with the same number. When I called him he said he didn't have a dog and had never heard of a Gil Gore."

"What are you trying to say?"

"I think we have a bogus, a cheat, a nonpayer."

"What about the address?"

"Well, now that I think about it, look at this. 210 38th Street. There isn't such a place. The last street east of here is 26th. If there was a 38th it would be out by the Martin Road. Come to think of it, when I asked him for his address and phone number, he hesitated as if he had to think about it. He screwed us. He had no intention of paying."

"I bet his name isn't Gill Gore either."

Rachel slapped the counter, "I should have gotten his truck license."

"We never learn do we Rachel," Alton commented with a little disappointment and sadness in his voice. "Am I that naïve Rachel? Am I that much of a sucker? An easy target? Every time someone says 'money is not a problem, do whatever it takes' I get left holding the bag."

"Don't beat up on yourself, Dr. Fried, your problem is not that you can be taken in but that you are just too kind and compassionate. You would have done exactly what you did for that dog even if you had known beforehand that you wouldn't get a penny for it."

"Yeah, I guess you're right," he said with a sigh.

"Most hospitals require a small amount in advance for first-time-clients, you don't even do that."

"Yes, but like in this case, if it's an emergency and the person has no money, what do you do?" He asked not expecting a reply.

"I know, your first concern is the animal."

"The dog can't help it if its owner is a crook. He'll love him til the end. Chalk up another one Rachel. See you bright and early; I'm going home."

TWENTY THREE

Dr. Friedson was alone in the hospital; Rachel had gone to the office supply store and Dr. Branberg was at the Kiwanis noon meeting presenting a talk on his trip to Mexico. He was a good, interesting speaker and when given a captive audience he could be very entertaining.

Alton picked up the phone on the first ring and didn't recognize the voice until the caller had mumbled a few sentences. He then realized it was John Wallace. John was a heavy smoker and drinker and when he had been too much into the bottle, his speech became a little difficult to understand. Even though it was only noon, it sounded like John was well on his way to a happy afternoon.

John was not a closet drinker. He liked his whiskey and he didn't care who knew it or what they thought about it. He would explain it by saying, "I have only two vices and I plan to enjoy them both to the fullest until I go broke or die – whichever comes first." His favorite brand was Jack Daniels Kentucky Bourbon, which he drank straight from the bottle with out a mixer. He couldn't imagine spoiling the smooth, rich taste of a good drink by diluting it with mixes or contaminated water. Before moving to the area he had worked for years at a Jack Daniels Distillery just outside of Lawrenceburg, Kentucky, near Lexington. It was there he had developed a taste for the drink and had been a loyal consumer and promoter ever since.

John lived by himself on his little farm and as far as anyone knew he was single and had no children. The only reference he ever made to women in Alton's presence was one late afternoon when they were together in a stall, and John was pretty tipsy. He had his arms wrapped lovingly around a horse's neck and said in a pensive voice, "Yah know, Doc, why would anyone wanna have a woman when he can have a horse. I can come out here any time I want and enjoy the company of one of my mares. Brush her sleek silken hair, rub her soft, warm skin, look into her big, beautiful brown eyes, feel her warm breath on my neck and not have to listen to her complain, bitch and nag twenty-four hours a day."

John hired himself out as a handyman and made a few dollars a week doing odd jobs around the community. The quality of his work was suspect, but the people he worked for were satisfied and paid him accordingly. A standing comment amongst his friends was that if you hire John, you better get him before noon because after twelve the quality of his work dips down as the bottle tips up.

John's farm was situated along the Stillaguamish River with enough pasture to adequately keep no more than four horses. The only problem with the location was that it lay on the lowest ground along the Bryant road, and when the river was high it usually flooded John's farm. John had three thoroughbred mares and gave them expert care, which he learned while working off and on at breeding farms in Kentucky. He knew when he needed the services of a vet and didn't hesitate to call.

He didn't introduce himself, just started right in, "Hey, Doc, 'member when I talked tu yah at the gas station. Told yah my mare wasn't eating good."

"Yeah, John, I remember. You said you'd call," Alton replied.

"Well, I'm calling. Now she's drooling a fair bit and turns her head to the side when she chews, like it hurts her jaws."

While John was talking, Alton heard the bell on the front door tinkle and heard someone walk to the front desk. He covered the mouth piece with his hand and in a loud voice said, "I'm on the phone; I'll be out in a minute.

John continued on, "Looks like she's dropping some weight, I can see her back ribs and with fall getting in I need to put some flesh on her. She seems to chomp the grass okay but has trouble with the alfalfa. Every morning ..."

Alton knew this conversation could go on for longer than he cared to listen, so he interrupted and said, "Listen, John, I have some free time this afternoon so I can run out. I'll be there in an hour or so. No need to keep her tied in, we'll get her when I get there." Without waiting for a reply he hung up the phone and walked out to the waiting room.

The man waiting for assistance was Mark Toomey, a good friend and a steady client.

"Hi, Alton," he said, extending his hand, "I was hoping you would be in."

"I'm the only one here. Sorry to keep you waiting. Got a problem? Don't tell me Missy's been eating rocks again," he said with a short laugh.

"No, I hope she's gotten over that. It's her mouth. It has a terrible smell and she keeps moving her tongue like she's chewing but she has no food."

"Is there any salivating or pawing at the face?" Alton asked.

"No. The most obvious thing is the smell. Like she ate something rotten and she's burping it up from her stomach," he answered.

"What is she now, Mark, six months?"

"She'll be eight in a couple of weeks."

"Still a puppy, and being a Lab she will stay a puppy for several years. Still chewing on everything I suppose."

"Everything she can get her mouth around," he laughed.

Alton started walking towards the surgery while motioning

to Mark's car. "Bring Missy in and put her on the table; it will only take a minute and I won't even charge you."

With Missy on the table and her head at eye level, Dr. Friedson lifted her upper lip and after a short whiff wrinkled his nose and said, "Whew, yup I've smelled that before."

"Nothing serious I hope," Mark asked.

"You'll see," Alton answered as he took a pair of forceps from his shirt pocket and, holding Missy by the back of her head, slowly inserted the instrument into the side of her mouth and along the hard palate until he hit something firm. "Just as I thought," he said. He opened the forceps, pushed a little harder, squeezed the handles, gave a short tug, and came out of the mouth holding a short stick of wood.

"Is this something like you were smelling?" he joked as he pushed the stick into Mark's face.

Mark covered his nose and pushed Dr. Friedson's hand aside. "How did you know that was there?" he seemed impressed.

"It all adds up," Dr. Friedson was giving Missy a quick going over as he talked. "Here's a young dog that likes to chew. She bites down on a stick and the sharp teeth snap it off on both ends and it gets lodged between the back molars. She keeps licking with her tongue but she can't get it out. Food and saliva get soaked into the wood and soon you have that putrid odor. I would guess this happened two or three days ago. It takes that long for the smell to get this strong."

"Poor girl, Missy, I didn't know," Mark shook her head between his hands.

"She'll be fine," Dr. Friedson said as he stepped out of the room.

"You said you wouldn't charge me, but there has to be something - if not for your time at least for your knowledge and expertise," Mark stood with his arms spread.

"Nope! Take her to the river for a run, she'll like that." He laughed as he said, "Give her a mint patty and squirt some Listerine in her mouth before you do any smooching."

Mark rolled his eyes and took the dog out the door.

TWENTY FOUR

Alton leaned on the top board of the fence as he watched the sleek, bay thoroughbred mare chew and swallow the late thinning grass in the pasture near the barn. Her head and jaw movements weren't normal, and he immediately concluded that she had a tooth problem.

When horses graze, they rarely lift their head. They can bite off the grass, chew, and swallow simultaneously and keep their nose to the ground for hours. If the grass is short or thin, they may lift their heads a little as they move from patch to patch. Otherwise, if they are hungry, it's nose to the ground.

As Alton stood watching, he thought how amazing the difference between the anatomy of the mouth and eating habits of the horse and the cow. Both are highly domestic animals with basically the same diet yet extremely different means in ingesting and digesting their food.

Horses have twelve sharp front teeth called incisors, six on the top jaw and six on the bottom. Cows have incisors only on the bottom jaw and none on the top. Horses bite, cows don't. Because of this, horses can bite off grass very close to the dirt and can survive on a small piece of ground if the grass grows rapidly. Cows are less fortunate. Because they can't bite, they take in grass by wrapping their tongue around the blades and cutting it off with their lower teeth. Thus the grass has to be quite long and it takes more ground to adequately feed a cow.

A horse chews and swallows its food as it keeps biting off more grass and taking it into its mouth. The horse has only one stomach, so once the grass is swallowed into the stomach it stays there and digestion begins. The cow is a ruminant, meaning it has four stomachs and an entirely different digestive system. When grass is taken into the mouth it stays there until a wad is formed, then it is swallowed into the first stomach, called the rumen. This continues until the cow decides she has had enough or some unforeseen circumstances force her to quit grazing. When the opportunity arises, she will lie down and quietly begin the digestive process.

She regurgitates a bolus of grass up through the esophagus and into her mouth, where she chews it, (referred to as chewing her cud), reswallows it and passes it into the second stomach, called the abomasum. From there it passes through the third and fourth stomachs before entering into the small intestine - a much different process than that of the horse.

One might wonder why nature would put such a complicated system into one of her animals, but there is a very logical reason. She slipped up when providing the cow with an inadequate means of protection from her predators, so she had to compensate for it. A cow can't run very fast, it can't bite, it doesn't have a very swift, hard kick, and some don't have horns. Its only good means of protection is to hide. So she goes out on the open plain in broad daylight, quickly fills her belly, then retreats to the upper ground, lies down and hides. There, in her quiet and safety, she can chew her cud and get on with the digestive process.

Unlike the cow and all other domestic animals, the teeth of the horse grow for the life of the horse from the time they erupt through the gums until the horse dies. In some aspects it is an asset as it allows the horse to repair damaged teeth, but it is also a tremendous liability because the teeth need attention periodically.

A more serious problem arises when a horse loses one or more of its molars. The corresponding tooth on the opposite jaw has no resistance so it continues to grow and eventually fills the hole in the opposite jaw. This also prohibits the teeth from grinding the food properly, and problems result. In this case the long growing tooth has to be cut off periodically, much to the discomfort of the uncooperative horse.

The one positive thing most horse owners can derive from this growing tooth phenomenon is that it is relatively easy to age a horse according to how the surfaces of the teeth wear. At certain ages the grinding surfaces and the shapes of the teeth change in such a way that a good horseman can come within six months of judging a horse's age. It is not fool-proof because of the horse's eating habits, but it is a good indicator.

John put a halter on the mare, led her into the barn and snapped her into the cross ties. There she would be adequately restrained for Dr. Friedson to do his examination. The two things he noticed first without even touching the mare, were a strong foul odor to her breath and a small swelling just below the left eye.

As he was putting a soft cotton glove on his left hand he turned to John and said, "Hey John, have you noticed anything unusual about her breath lately?"

"About her breath? No. Except that she is breathing," he started to laugh, and then ended up bent over with his hands on his knees and coughing like he wanted to spit up.

Alton reached in with his gloved hand and took hold of the mare's tongue pulled it sideways out of her mouth and pushed it back between her back teeth. This would prevent her from closing her mouth, providing Dr. Friedson digital access to the rear molars. He ran his fingers along the upper molars feeling their sharp edges, and when he got to the last tooth the mare flinched - not much, but enough that Alton noticed it. He paused for a moment then pushed on it a little harder. There was definitely some pain there. He finished examining the other arcades, released the horse's tongue, then stepped back and took off the glove. John was sitting on a water bucket with a bottle of whiskey on his lap.

"Whatcha find Doc, a piece of wire or something? I thought she may have a stick or a rock caught in a tooth." John didn't get up, just sat hunched over with his back pressed against the stall door.

"She has an abscessed tooth John, and one of the worst ones to get to. I think it has been bad for awhile because the sinus is infected; she has a swelling in the maxillary sinus just below her left eye."

"Just give her a shot of penicillin. Shoot, she's a tough old gal. She'll recover and be as good as new," he said, waving the bottle at the horse.

"Untie her and take her to a dry patch of grass in the field away from the other horses. I'll get the things I need."

John fumbled with the ropes as he held the bottle in one hand. Alton slapped him on the shoulder and said, "Leave that bottle here. We have work to do!"

"Damn it, Doc, you're not my mother!" He slammed the bottle on the water bucket and led the horse towards the door.

"By the way, what's her name?" Dr. Friedson called after him.

"Her papered handle is Roseinthemorn. Her sire's name was Upandatem and her dam's name was Roseinbloom. I call her my dear Rosie."

Pounding out and cutting off a horse's rear molar is not an easy job. The horse is anesthetized, laid on its side and a clumsy metal contraption called a speculum is placed in the mouth and cranked open as far as possible for access to the rear molars.

To make sure he had made the right diagnosis, Alton wiggled

the molar with a large pair of forceps and watched as puss oozed out from the gum line. The tooth had to come out.

He cut a two-inch hole in the skin just below the left eye, and then drilled a hole through the facial bone to expose the sinus. He flushed away the exudate until he could see the root of the infected tooth. He took a metal punch, placed it on the root, and with a heavy hammer, gave it a few hard whacks. After the third blow he felt the tooth loosen and give a little. He continued to tap on it until the tooth was protruding about an inch and resting on the tooth of the lower jaw. He then took a long-handled pair of dental side cutters and cut about an inch off the tooth. He again hit on the root of the tooth until it was resting on the lower tooth, and again he cut it off. He continued this until he was able to pull the remaining root from the cavity, leaving a gaping hole through the jaw and into the sinus.

The next step was to plug the hole so hay and grain wouldn't be pushed up into the sinus cavity. He took a long piece of suture tape and tied it to a large wad of gauze. Threading the tape through the jaw, he pulled the gauze into the hole and packed it tight with his fingers. He left the tape hanging from the sinus to use when changing the gauze plug. He poured a mild iodine solution into the sinus, gave Rosie 20cc's of penicillin-streptomycin, and then leaned back on his heels.

As he was gathering up his equipment, he said, "I'll stay with her until she is on her feet, then I'll come back in two days to see how she is doing and change that plug." He looked over at John for some kind of reply, but there wasn't going to be one. John was sprawled out on the ground with his back pressed against Rosie's belly, face turned to the sun, fast asleep.

TWENTY FIVE

I t seemed this was going to be a week responding to horse calls. The schedule between horses and cows seemed to run in cycles. There would be several days when Alton would run from morning til night to keep up with the horse appointments, and then there would be times when there were more dairy calls. He was pleased that the horse business was picking up because his long-range plans were to someday have his own practice, limited to horses and built around a modern equine hospital. With each call he made he felt his dream becoming closer to reality. He was gaining confidence and knowledge in both working with and treating horses, and building a clientele that had faith in his judgment, abilities and medical expertise. He was getting referrals not only from regular clients but also from those who had called him for the first time. He had to admit he got a little puffed up when complimented on a difficult case or when someone spoke highly of him as an equine doctor. He felt comfortable around the horses and had a feeling that the horses bonded quickly to his gentle voice and soft touch.

Through the information gained from books, veterinary journals, case write-ups, seminars, and conventions Alton was confident he could successfully manage most routine problems he would encounter at the local farms. However, there were times when he had to shrug his shoulders and say, "I don't know." Often the owner of the horse would offer a suggestion or tell of an old treatment his dad or grandfather had used years ago. This happened to Alton at the Slotten farm one summer afternoon.

Emily Slotten called to say she didn't have an emergency but her daughter's horse, Mermaid, was acting a little strange and probably should be looked at soon. If Dr. Friedson was in the area, she would appreciate it if I would stop in. The problem with that statement was they lived eighteen miles east of town along the South River Highway, not even close to one of his regular clients. It could be days before he was out that way, and the horse's condition could be serious by then. He decided to make it a single call even though Mrs. Slotten would have to pay for the fifteen dollar trip charge.

Mermaid was standing in the shade of a growth of alders when Alton and Mrs. Slotten approached the paddock. She didn't attempt to move and didn't raise her head or whinny to greet them. Emily pointed to the horse and said, "Now you see, this is not normal. If she were okay, she would be up to this fence in a flash looking for a handout or a pat on the neck."

"Is she an affectionate type of horse?" Alton asked.

"Oh, she loves people and prances and acts up when someone comes. In fact, that's what caused the injury last week."

"What kind of an injury?"

"Last week Jennifer had some friends here for a sleepover, and they were out running around acting up and got Mermaid all excited. She reared up next to that board fence over there, and when she came down she caught her fetlock on a nail on the post. The girls noticed the blood but the hole was so small we didn't do anything about it. Then yesterday we noticed she seemed a little stiff, so maybe her leg is hurting her more than we thought."

"Can we get to her?" he asked, looking around for a gate.

"I can put her in the barn."

"No, I would prefer walking up to her and observing her reaction."

"Yeah, we can go through the back door of the barn," she said, pointing the way.

As they walked through the barn, Alton was thinking of three possible diagnoses: Tetanus, a terribly sore foot, or a very high temperature. All three would make the horse listless and reluctant to move. First he would rule out an abnormally high temperature because he could do that easily and quickly.

Tetanus in a horse is easy to diagnose because there are no other conditions that give all the similar telltale symptoms. If there has been a recent injury and the doctor knows a few of the simple tests, there is no excuse to not diagnose this condition.

When Alton approached the horse, he ran his hand along the neck under the mane, then down her face and over her nose, then reached up and felt her ears. He slowly slid his hand into her mouth and gently wrapped his hand around her tongue. He estimated her temperature to be 100 degrees – normal for a horse.

He took a hold of her halter to lead her forward, and she did walk but with some difficulty and a very stiff gait. This was not due to a sore foot. He dropped the halter, walked in front of Mermaid and motioned for Emily to stand still and be quiet. He then clapped his hands hard and loud in front of Mermaid's face, looking her straight in the eye as he did so. He saw what he expected. The third eyelid, the nictitating membrane, shot across the eyeball covering it for just a second with the thin membrane. Alton waited a moment, then repeated the clap with the same result. That was one positive diagnostic test for tetanus.

He took hold of the halter with both hands and gently moved the head from side to side, then downward, but when he tried to lift it up, the horse resisted, tensed her neck muscles and appeared very uncomfortable: another positive sign for tetanus.

He walked around the horse, lifting each leg and finding them firm and stiff and difficult to bend. Mermaid acted as if she might fall down if all four feet were not planted firmly on the ground - another sign of tetanus.

The last test, the movement of the jaws would confirm the diagnosis. The layman's term for tetanus is lockjaw because a person or animal with tetanus finds it difficult to open their mouth. The maxillary muscles of the jaws are in a permanent state of contraction, preventing the mouth from being able to open.

Alton could not entice Mermaid to open her jaws or spread them apart with his hands. She really didn't object to him trying; she just stood quietly seemingly unconcerned about what he was doing.

"I'm positive she has an advanced case of tetanus," he said, dropping his hands to his side and giving Emily a sad look.

"That's fatal in horses, isn't it?" She knew the answer before she asked it.

"I have not had one survive, even having done everything we could think of. They'll live awhile but without being able to eat or drink, they deteriorate rapidly."

"I am sure Jennifer will want to try. She'll follow instructions to the letter. She loves this mare."

"There really isn't a lot that can be done. No physical labor. The hardest part is the waiting and making the decision whether or not to put her down if it comes to that. If we are going to try to save her, we have to start right now."

Mrs. Slotten dug her hands into her pockets and said, "So they still haven't found a cure for this yet. What causes tetanus, anyway?"

"It is caused by a specific germ, the bacillus tetani that gets into the blood and produces a chemical poison that irritates the nervous system, causing muscular contractions and cramps. The organisms enter the body through an injury, and because they do better without oxygen, they like deep puncture wounds like those caused by a nail or other long, sharp object. It probably entered through the puncture wound in Mermaid's fetlock."

"The vaccine tetanus toxoid can be given to prevent the condition, but it has to be given once a year and Mermaid probably didn't get one recently. Time flies by." He didn't want Emily to feel guilty, but he wanted her to have the information.

"So what do we do now? Jennifer will be home from school soon. Should we wait til she gets here so you can explain it to her?"

"Let's try to get Mermaid into the barn and settled in. Your daughter should be here by then."

The instructions, what to look for, and what to expect, given to Emily and Jennifer were detailed and specific.

"Mermaid must be kept in an absolute dark and quiet stall, no exceptions. Noise makes the condition worse because the muscles tend to tighten more. Only one person should tend to her to avoid stress and confusion, and when in the stall that person should move slowly and talk in whispers. Mermaid will not eat but may drink a little if the bucket is on the floor. She will not want to raise her head or lie down. You must keep her on her feet. If she does go down, she will be unable to get up. Even though she may sweat profusely, keep her blanketed at all times with a cooler sheet, which can be changed, and a good but light blanket. She will appear to be in pain and agony at all times because of the wide eyes, flared nostrils and heavy breathing, but it is more muscle tension than pain. Most horses with an advanced case won't live more than three weeks, but if they get past nine days a big percentage will make it. I will clean the wound and give an antibiotic, but other than that there is no medication available to help her along."

Jennifer had a long, sad face. "Is there the least bit of chance she will live, Dr. Friedson?" she asked.

"I'm extremely sympathetic, Jennifer, but her chances are very slim. My experience tells me she is probably not going to make it. I'm sorry."

As Alton was putting his things away, he didn't notice that Emily had followed him out to the truck.

"I didn't want to say anything with Jennifer present because I didn't want her to get her hopes up," Emily said. "I may have something to try. You will probably think I have lost all my marbles but it is worth mentioning."

"Anything that will help is worth listening to," Alton replied.

"I have an aunt in California who peddles herself as an herb specialist and healer. I heard her mention once about a plant she had that could cure the strangest of diseases. I distinctly heard her say it will even cure tetanus. I could call her and get more information and find out what it's about."

"I'm up to trying anything," he said as he opened the door to the truck. "Give me a call. We don't have much time."

When Alton walked into the hospital, he heard Rachel on the phone. "I'll tell him when he gets in, Mrs. Slotten, I'm sure he will be pleased to hear there is something that can be done."

"Did she get in touch with her aunt?" he asked.

"Yes and her aunt was very optimistic. She is sending a package by air mail, including instructions on how to prepare an herb tea and how to administer it. The post office will call Mrs. Slotten and she will have you pick it up and take it with you to the farm. This will be a new notch in your belt."

"I hate it when people are given false hope with some miracle medicine when most of the time it just prolongs the animal's suffering, debilitation and eventual death. But we'll do what she says, and the Slottens will know they did all they could." He went into his office and reached for the phone to call his wife.

To Alton's surprise it was less than 48 hours later that Mrs. Slotten called to ask him to pick up the package at the post office and hurry out to the farm. Mermaid was holding her own but getting visibly weaker, and she was afraid Mermaid might go down. Maybe the herbal tea might have time to work

The box contained a bag of leaves and twigs resembling alfalfa with a faint minty smell. The instructions were simple. Put one-third of the leaves in 6 quarts of near-boiling water for 15 minutes, then let it steep for 30 minutes. Drain off the leaves and let the tea cool. Make three similar batches. Administer 2 quarts orally every 4 hours for 36 hours. Some improvement should be visible within 18 to 24 hours. If there is no change after 36 hours, then the medicated tea didn't work.

Mermaid offered little resistance when Alton passed the plastic tube through her nose and into her stomach and poured 2 quarts of the tea into the funnel. He tied the tube to Mermaid's halter so Jennifer could use it to administer the rest of the medication at 4 hour intervals. Now it was just a matter of time. He hoped the concoction would have some effect because the horse was rapidly getting worse.

When the phone rang Alton said, "Oh, no," when he looked at the clock and saw it was only six in the morning. Rolling over, he thought, "Not an emergency this early." He picked up the receiver and barely said hello when an excited voice interrupted him, "Dr. Friedson, we think she is getting better! Her breathing is better, her nostrils are smaller, her head is up a little and her tail is pressed tight against her buttocks. She might make it!"

Alton sat straight up in bed, "Jennifer that is terrific news. You had no trouble getting the tea into her?"

"Oh no, we couldn't get her head up very high but we got it all into the tube and into her stomach. I am so excited, I am sure she is going to make it."

"So now you have three treatments left, is that right? You should be done at six tonight." He figured that would be a total of nine.

"Yes," she replied. "Do you think you could come up tonight and check her? I think you will be surprised."

"I'll be there in time to help with the treatment, then I can take the tube out. I'll see you then."

The case of the backyard pleasure horse with an advanced case of tetanus was one for the books: a typical rusty nail puncture wound, definite diagnostic symptoms of tetanus, a pessimistic prognosis, and then a miraculous recovery using an unheard of, nonmedically-approved herbal tea.

Mermaid made a one hundred percent complete recovery with no after-effects. Dr. Friedson never did learn the name of the herb, but he made a mental memo of where he could get it if he ever needed it again.

The whole scenario was a perfect example of how a so-called "snake oil" could outwrestle medical science to give a creature new life and bring happiness to a destitute family.

TWENTY SIX

Before leaving for home, Dr. Friedson usually checked the next day's work schedule so he could prepare himself and stock his car for the first calls the following morning. This night he had gone straight home from his last farm call so wasn't aware of his first few calls when he arrived at the hospital just before 8:00 a.m. When he looked at the books and saw he was scheduled to be at the Robert's farm he knew it wasn't going to be a pleasant morning.

"Rachel, why didn't you tell me you scheduled Roberts for this morning?" he called out from his office.

"Why? So you could call in sick!" she replied.

"That or just keep heading north into Canada."

"Get over it. He pays his bill on time each month and we need the money."

"Yeah, but when I get through with him my psychiatry bill is higher than his vet account. I'm losing ground. Maybe today won't be too traumatic. I see he just wants the colts dewormed and given their second round of shots."

Glen Roberts had only two permanent farm horses – two older, decently bred thoroughbred mares. Each spring he bred them both to local studs, always got them pregnant and had two early foals. He sold them privately as yearlings to local buyers and was fortunate enough to get a few to the race track and even record a win now and then.

His best mare, Paddycakes, was a seventeen-hand chestnut by Succession, who stood at the Machias Stables and at one time was considered to be the top stud in the state. Paddycakes had the breeding to produce some high- powered offspring but Glen Roberts was too cheap to spend the money to breed her to a top-notch stud. Many of the mare's foals were purchased for hunter jumpers and dressage performers. They were popular because of their size and agility.

The other broodmare was smaller, dark brown with a narrow blaze running from her forelock to her upper lip. She was named Earlybirdy by Glen's wife because she was born on January second. Her sire was Mister Mustard, whose son Mustard Plaster was a big money winner at Longacres. Earlybirdy's foals were usually small, fine-boned and more refined than most sturdy thoroughbreds. They looked more like Arabians than racing thoroughbreds. Her foals were popular with members of the local Pony Clubs because they were good-looking and superior athletes.

Glen Roberts was a very impatient man with no time for extraneous conversation or wasted minutes. He always appeared to be in a hurry and didn't hesitate to express his displeasure if Dr. Friedson was late or unprepared, or if procedures didn't go to his liking.

Before leaving the hospital Alton checked his equipment and supplies to be sure he had everything he needed so Mr. Roberts would have no reason to criticize: deworming medication, tubes, clean water pail, lubricant, vaccines, syringes, clean boots and overalls. He made sure he had his nose clamp twitch, as Glen would not tolerate the use of a chain twitch. He considered it to be cruel and inhumane. Both he and Alton welcomed the metal squeeze twitch, which was effective but wasn't painful.

"I'm off," Alton shouted, "if I'm not back by noon send out the search party."

"You know if you didn't think so bad of him things might go better for you," Rachel replied encouragingly.

"Well, if the odds are with me I might have a good one."

He slipped out the back door and headed the blue Ford north on the old highway, determined not to be late. When he arrived at the farm Mr. Roberts was leading the two weanlings into the barn, an old cement block structure that Glen had converted into six stalls and a space for hay storage. The shavings were kept outside in a wooden bunker covered with a heavy blue tarp that flapped in the wind, allowing rain to blow in and soak the chips.

"Good morning, Dr. Friedson." He was always friendly and cheerful when Alton was on time. "I want the two babies dewormed for strongyles and ascarids and have their second influenza and distemper shots. I want the yearlings up-to-date on their medical records. I am considering sending the Captain Courageous colt to the Summer Sale. I also want you to check and see if the mares are due for a Rhino shot."

"Are you sure you want the young ones to have a distemper shot?" Dr. Friedson asked.

"Yeah, I don't want them to be all swollen and snotty, off their feed, losing weight and looking rough when the inspectors come. Besides, it takes them months to recover."

"As you know, it's only a bacterin, Glen, and not 100% effective. I think sometimes foals get the symptoms from the shot. The bug has to be transmitted by contact, and you are pretty much isolated out here. If you are careful who comes on the place and who handles the boys, I don't think you should have a problem."

"I want the works." Glen said without hesitating.

Alton knew it was a lost cause to try to convince him to reconsider.

They started by vaccinating the mares for Rhinotracheitis, a contagious virus which often caused abortion in pregnant mares. They required one shot during each trimester of their pregnancy.

Deworming and vaccinating the two yearlings went well because, by now, they had been handled and worked with several times and were disciplined to respect the nose clamp. Alton commented on how great the Captain colt looked. He was tall, sleek, muscular and well-balanced with a long neck, smooth withers, and strong hind quarters. He could do well at the sale.

Alton knew the weanlings could be a handful. They are just big enough and strong enough not to be restrained by a not-so-strong person and yet young enough not to know how to behave. Glen was not a big man, about five feet eight weighing around 150 pounds and a bit out of shape from sitting behind a desk for most of his working days. Another thing that didn't help the situation was something that Alton wouldn't divulge to anyone, but he had worked with Glen enough to suspect that he was actually afraid of horses. When one jumped or moved quickly, Glen jumped twice as high sending tack and equipment flying.

Having a rubber hose pushed up through the nose is an unwelcome surprise for a weanling who has not experienced such mistreatment in his or her traumatic-free, short life. The filly or colt is haltered, backed into a corner of the stall and a metal clamp is squeezed over the delicate, soft tissue of the upper lip. Then, as if it understands the English language, the horse is told to stand still. Better yet, the weanling is told that when the twitch is on the nose, that is a time to behave and be quiet. But of course some take longer than others for this to sink in.

The procedure is quick and simple and takes only a few minutes if all goes well and according to plan. Alton approaches the horse from the right side and slowly passes the lubricated tube into the right nostril, over the pharynx, down the esophagus and into the stomach. The medication is poured into a funnel at the end of the tube and runs into the stomach and intestines, where it effectively kills the nasty parasites that have taken up housekeeping.

Surprisingly, the first colt took the tightening of the halter and the pressure of the twitch quite well and stood quietly while Dr. Friedson put his left hand on the colt's nose and began inserting the tube into his nostril. All was well until he felt the end of the tube pressing against the turbinates in the nose and the colt decided this was no longer fun. He shook his head vigorously from side to side, and Dr. Friedson's heart stopped. He heard the turbinates crack, felt the tearing of the tissues and he knew that soon the blood would come gushing, and once it started it wouldn't stop. The blood vessels of the nose are thin, close to the surface and when ruptured, a serious nose bleed is in the making.

At this point, although it is bloody and messy, there is no quitting. The colt has to be dewormed and the only recourse is to keep poking and pushing until the tube passes regardless of the trauma and blood loss.

The more Dr. Friedson pushed and twisted the tube, the more the colt shook his head, pawed the ground, and snorted through his nose, and blood was everywhere. Mr. Roberts was totally fatigued. He released the twitch, allowing the colt to leap into the air, knocking Glen to the floor and leaving Dr. Friedson standing with a scared look on his blood-spattered face and a bloody rubber tube hanging from his right hand.

Now in fairness to Dr. Friedson, it must be stated that tubing a weanling without drawing some blood is difficult to do. The rubber tube is not much smaller than the nostril and the blood vessels in the nose are very fragile. Most inexperienced veterinarians will induce a nose bleed more often than not. Because of Dr. Friedson's tenderness and experience he seldom got a nose bleed, but when it happens, as he will state, it always seems to be at the wrong place at the wrong time.

Mr. Roberts picked himself up from the floor, his face bright red, partly from internal rage and partly from the bleeding nose of his prized colt.

"What's the matter with you?" he shouted. "Now look what you've done." He tried to steady himself against the wall. "You idiot, haven't you wormed a colt before? How do you get off passing yourself off as a veterinarian? You've probably ruined one of my best colts. You call yourself a horse vet? Who are you trying to kid?" He walked over to Alton and poked a finger into his face. "I should report you, you quack. Talk about an incompetent piece of work, boy, you sure are one! I've seen some shoddy, sloppy, unprofessional work but you sure set the standard."

Dr. Friedson stood and listened for awhile, slowly coiled the tube and put it in the pail along with the twitch, the medication and the lubricant, then walked over to check the colt's bleeding nose.

"What do you think you are doing? Where do you think you are going?" Glen yelled, stepping in front of Alton. "You haven't finished the job here, mister. You're responsible."

Dr. Friedson didn't say a word, just walked out of the stall and towards the large door at the end of the alleyway.

"Listen to me, Friedson, if you don't come back and finish this it will be the end of your career, such as it is, I promise you!"

Dr. Friedson stopped, turned to face Mr. Roberts and in a slow, quiet voice said, "Mr. Roberts, I'm leaving. Your verbal abuse and accusations are embarrassing, insulting and intolerable. When you have exhausted all your attempts to get another equine veterinarian, or any veterinarian, to come to this barn, you will call me again. I have enjoyed working for you but, I am sorry to say, I won't be coming back. Goodbye."

Glen stood quietly, not speaking a word, a sorry sight with straw stuck to the drying blood covering his shirt and pants. He was struck dumb, realizing that what he had just heard was probably the gospel truth.

TWENTY SEVEN

While driving back to the hospital Alton couldn't decide whether to feel sad, mad, glad or all three. He was sad and sorry for the colt that had to experience the discomfort and frightening pressure of the twitch on his delicate upper lip and the strange feeling of a foreign object sliding up his nostril. The colt's reaction was normal and expected and the nose bleed was the result of his reaction. Though unpleasant, it was a common occurrence when tubing young horses with an inexperienced handler. The good thing is that there is no lasting damaging affect from the trauma.

Alton also felt mad and disappointed with Mr. Roberts for his reaction and tirade over an incident that Alton was sure he had experienced before with someone else, or at least heard that nose bleeds happen. His harsh words were hurtful – "Pretending to be a vet; ruining my best colt; you idiot; you quack; you incompetent piece of work." Alton was not deserving of such treatment. He thought back and said out loud to himself, "I have done Glen's horse work for at least three years. I have tube dewormed three sets of weanlings and yearling three times a year, plus the mares several times, all without drawing a drop of blood - a pretty darn good track record." There was no excuse for Glen's behavior and it made Alton more upset the more he thought about it.

Alton may have been glad to have lost a client who had a tendency to cause undue stress and be a trouble-maker. His trips to the farm always seemed to cause some sort of irritability, which he didn't need and certainly didn't want. Glen was like fingernails on the black board - irritating but harmless. Alton's horse practice was growing steadily and was getting to the point where he had the privilege to pick and choose. If there was a potential irritant in the mix he had the right and the pleasure to remove it.

He needed a distraction and remembering the day was Tuesday, he shifted his thoughts to the Jaycee dinner and meeting he would attend later in the evening.

TWENTY EIGHT

Alton was president of the active Chapter 7 of the Washington State Jaycees, a civic organization of young men between the ages of 18 and 37 dedicated to the betterment of their community. They used their time, talents, skills, and monies to participate in community programs and projects to assist in making their cities a better, safer and more pleasant place to live and work.

Chapter 7 consisted of 64 energetic, young men and Alton always looked forward to the weekly meetings to share and participate in the camaraderie, laughter, project planning, and lively discussions that took place when they got together. There were annual projects that needed chairpersons, workers, organizing, and planning. The Fourth of July fireworks stand, the Tulip Festival Salmon Barbecue, the County Fair Parade, the Christmas street decorations, the Skagit River Raft Race, and assisting other civic organizations with some of their community programs.

Alton was proud of his membership in the Jaycees and felt he was a good, hardworking, and successful leader. The local club thought so too because at their annual Fall Awards Banquet they presented him with The Distinguished Service Award given to the young man whom the chapter considered had been an outstanding member and had given unselfishly to the betterment of the community.

Of all the accolades given him during his time in the Chapter, the one Alton cherished most was being voted in by his peers as a

Washington State Jaycee Governor - the highest award presented to a Jaycee. He was the first member from Chapter 7 to receive the award, which was presented to him at the State Convention held in Yakima. It was a humbling experience to say the least.

TWENTY NINE

As Alton drove down the driveway to the big two-story country home, he noticed Alice and Marie sitting on the old metal swing in the back yard. The ponies Martha and Dippidy were standing next to the fence hoping the girls would have a carrot or an apple for an evening treat. Alton stepped out of the car and walked across the yard.

"Good evening ladies, need a push?" He asked.

"Yes," Marie shouted, "but I want on the saddle seats so we can go real high." She scrambled from the swing chair to the little board seat. Alton walked behind her and started pushing. She screamed with delight yelling, "higher, higher." But Alton knew the limit. The swing wasn't fastened to the ground and if the girls swung too fast and too high the legs of the swing could lift up and tip over. When the swing slowed he said, "I think it must be time for supper. Better get washed up. Race you to the door."

Allan was practicing a song on the piano and Bev was busy in the kitchen. When Ann saw her dad walk in she pushed herself up onto her feet and began climbing on the top rail of her play pen and making baby noises. She was a good baby and why she was content to remain in her play pen for most of the day was a mystery but certainly good for Bev who had more to do than hold and watch a baby all day.

Alton wondered how Bev did it every day. He was usually up early and on the road before the rest of the family was out of bed. Often he didn't get home til late. Because of this schedule, Bev was alone with the kids all day during the summer when there was no school. She had to dress them, feed them, bathe them, watch over them, and yes, reprimand them. When shopping or running errands they had to be dressed in clean clothes and shoes and kept within eyesight while trying to concentrate on what she was doing. Allan and Alice were old enough to be of some help but they were often distracted and not too dependable.

Alton tried to help as much as he could, especially with the kids, but there was the farm to look after and most of his time was spent in maintenance projects, gardening, fencing, caring for the animals, and the dozens of small jobs necessary to keep ahead of possible problems. He was a handyman, a good farmer and took pride in keeping the gardens weeded, the grass mowed, buildings painted and fences in good repair. Many times when he was busy in the yard or working with the horses he took the older kids with him to get them out of the house and give Bev a break.

One thing Bev had going for her was that there were several families in the area with kids the same age as Allan, Alice, and Marie. Within walking distance there were six families with two or more young children. Because the Friedsons had a large, flat yard, swings, bike trails, large trees, horses, a big old hay barn and access to the Nookachamps Creek, the locals used it as a playground and often gathered there to play their games or to just hang out. It served as a babysitting tool for Bev and gave her some private time to herself.

"Dean Mannak called," Bev said as she stirred what smelled like a pot of spaghetti, "He wanted to talk about your hunting trip."

"He's still planning to go I hope."

"He didn't say. He was calling from the hospital. Jean was having her knee X-rayed. It's been giving her trouble again."

"I think he wants to go without horses this year. Last year they gave us some trouble and they take a lot of care."

Dean Mannak and Alton had been classmates in medical

school and remained close friends after graduation. Alton was instrumental in getting Dean a position in a clinic eighty miles south of Mount Vernon; close enough for the two families to visit together.

Every year Dean and Alton went hunting deer, elk or pheasants and sometimes all three. This year they were planning an elk hunting trip in the Salmon River area in north central Idaho. As of yet, Dean had not shot an elk, but two years ago Alton bagged a nice five point bull on Bethel Ridge near Yakima. After walking and stalking for a couple of hours Alton decided to take a break and sat down by a spreading pine tree alongside a game trail. He closed his eyes to rest a moment and enjoy the quiet and familiar sounds of nature. When he opened them again he was startled and surprised to see three elk cows walking directly toward him on the trail, followed by a big bull elk. He dared not move; just sat and stared. His heart began to pound and his mind took off running. What to do? Elk are so perceptive and suspicious, not curious like a deer.

Assessing the situation, Alton figured he had two options; jump up quickly and hope to get a good shot, or move into position as slowly as possible and hope the sharp eyes of the bull didn't notice. With the first option he would have to wait until the herd was very close, within 50 yards. But at that range it was possible they could pick up his scent and bolt into the woods. If he was going to move slowly he would have to do it now in order to get his 7mm rifle into position without being noticed.

He decided on the second option – move slowly and take his chances. As he slowly moved his hand down to the butt of his rifle, the animals suddenly stopped as if they had seen something. Alton thought to himself 'how could they? My hand moved only six inches and they are 150 yards away'. They stood for awhile then the rear cow walked around the others and took a sharp turn moving up a small rise among some small pine trees. The others followed with the bull bringing up the rear.

Alton heaved a sigh of relief; what a break. This would be the perfect broadside shot. He picked a clearing about five yards wide between two trees where the elk would pass, raised his rifle, took sight, and waited. The first cow passed and Alton leveled on the chest just behind the right front leg. Then the second and third cows passed and Alton did the same sighting; practicing for the big moment. Then came the unsuspecting bull; proud beast of the herd. When he was perfectly framed between the two trees Alton slowly squeezed the trigger, there was a sharp crack and the bull staggered to the ground.

It took a half day to get the carcass dressed, quartered, and carried back to camp. The rack of horns is proudly displayed on the wall in Alton's downstairs den.

THIRTY

"Well, you know what I think of your specialist," Mr. Pierson said in a harsh voice that expressed his disappointment.

"You said he was the best sheep doctor in Canada, and he killed my best ewe. Tell him to go back to where he came from."

Mr. Pierson was quite upset because he had been assured that his sick ewe was in good medical care when he brought her in to the hospital, and he had gone home thinking she would be okay and he could pick her up in a couple of days. She was his favorite of all the ewes in his herd of Dorset sheep, and he had rushed her into the hospital when he thought she might die.

Doctor Rand Branberg, the owner of the Valley Animal Hospital, was a practical joker and when Mr. Pierson called to say he had a very sick ewe, Dr. Branberg seized the opportunity to have a little fun with his farmer friend. A brother-in-law of Dr. Branberg's associate, Dr. Alton Friedson, was visiting for a few days and happened to be standing in the hospital when the call came in. Dr. Branberg whooped a little and said, "So you have a sick ewe do you, well this must be your lucky day, Jon, we just happen to have a sheep specialist from Canada visiting for a few days and he could look at your ewe this afternoon. Bring her right in and put her in the big dog run and I'll have the good doctor get right to her when he and Dr. Friedson return from taking their lunch."

He chuckled as he hung up the phone, but Rachel thought it was a long way from a practical joke.

"You know what's going to happen, don't you," she said with a little bite to her words. "The sheep is going to die and poor Mr. Amsey is going to get blamed for it. He is a construction worker, for Pete's sake."

"Come on, Rachel, lighten up," he waved his arms and giggled. "We'll give the old sheep a shot of penicillin, she'll recover from her mild fever, Mr. Pierson will take her home and Mr. Amsey will be a hero. We'll all have a good laugh and Mr. Amsey will have a good story to tell his grandchildren."

"Don't count your chickens before they hatch," Rachel said, as she closed the door to the surgery.

When Dr. Friedson heard that Jon Pierson had trucked in a sick ewe, he was more than just a little concerned. It had to be a serious case for the poor farmer to spend a lot of money and time to take an animal to a hospital and not take care of the critter himself. Jon and Edna were scratching deep down to make a living on a run-down farm with poor quality soil and a variety of animals. They were capable of routine medical treatments and called a doctor only when the situation was beyond their expertise.

The Pierson farm could easily be taken for the county garbage dump. There hadn't been a building, fence, or piece of machinery repaired in years and it appeared that anything that could break or fall down had done so. It was almost impossible to walk or drive through the farm without tripping over or running into a pile of junk. Years of accumulation of metal, wire, glass, and boards occupied every accessible place around the house and barns, and wandering amongst this clutter and rubble was a variety of farm life to rival the county zoo. It was unbelievable that at least one of the goats, pigs, turkeys, ducks, chickens or dogs didn't injure or impale themselves while tiptoeing through and around the debris. Dr. Friedson was sure this is what had happened to the ewe that was being brought in.

Edna Pierson loved and cared for all the birds and animals on the farm except for the cows and sheep, which was the responsibility of her husband. The Piersons were a living imitation of Ma and Pa Kettle. Jon was tall and lanky, carrying about 130 pounds on a skeleton of a frame, slightly bent at the waist and rounded at the shoulders. He had a submissive personality and spoke with a guttural drawl so low in his throat that it was sometimes hard to understand him. He was a rather pitiful looking man, but he had a kind soul and loved his farm.

Edna, on the other hand, was large, round and definitely the ruler of the roost. When she shouted; everyone from the chicks in the brooder to the bull in the breed pen pricked their ears. She always wore a printed dress with a full length apron that had to be changed several times a day as it served as a basket for carrying eggs and injured chicks, a towel for wiping hands and a damp cloth for wiping weepy eyes and runny noses. Although she was big in stature and appeared to be coarse in nature, she had a soft voice and had a calming affect on the brood she attended to.

When Dr. Friedson and his brother-in-law, Stew Amsey, returned from lunch, Dr. Branberg was standing in the large dog run eyeing a very weak and sad looking Dorset ewe. As soon as they stepped into the run, Dr. Branberg started to laugh, slapped Stew on the back and said, "Well, Doctor Amsey, you've got your work cut out for you. I told Mr. Pierson we had a sheep specialist from Canada visiting today and you would have his prize ewe up and as good as new in no time. He went home delighted that his Bonnie was in the hands of an expert and that he would be able to pick her up in a couple of days." Mr. Amsey, going along with the prank, let out a weak laugh and said, "Well, everyone is entitled to fifteen minutes of fame during his lifetime."

Hearing the conversation, Rachel poked her head in the door

and shouted pessimistically, "Well you better save the critter or your Doctor Amsey won't get back across the border."

After reading a history of listlessness, abdominal cramps, lack of appetite and no feces for several days, the doctors agreed the problem was probably some form of intestinal obstruction. It was difficult to put their finger on a diagnosis because they could feel nothing definitive on abdominal palpation and their antiquated X-ray machine was not strong enough to get good diagnostic radiographs. After a short conference it was decided to do an exploratory laperotomy. Rachel was instructed to call the Piersons to get their permission and tell them one of the doctors would call as soon as the operation was completed.

The ewe was anesthetized while lying on the floor. Then Dr. Branberg held the ether mask over her nose while Stew and Alton lifted her onto the surgery table. Her belly was clipped, scrubbed three times with an iodine soap, then completely draped with surgical sheets. The instruments were laid on the side table and the light was adjusted to shine on the middle of the ewe's abdomen.

Dr. Friedson made a three inch incision just posterior to the umbilicus, and as some fluid oozed out onto the drape he dropped the scalpel and let out a loud sigh.

"Oh, no!"

"What?" asked Dr. Branberg, turning on the stool to look.

"The abdominal fluid is black and has texture," Dr. Friedson replied, rubbing some of the fluid between his fingers.

Dr. Branberg stood up and tilting his head so his bifocals were in focus, stared at the incision.

"It's got a necrotic smell. That's not good," he said, bending down for a closer look.

"Boy, that downright stinks," Stew said, squinching up his nose.

Looking at the coffee-colored fluid seeping from the incision and getting a good whiff of the foul smell, Dr. Friedson knew the prognosis even before he saw the condition of the abdominal tissues. He extended the incision caudally to the pubis, opened the belly and looked inside. His suspicions were verified when he saw the condition of the intestines and the color of the abdominal wall. It was obvious there was intestinal involvement with a puncture or rupture allowing ingesta to leak into the abdomen, causing peritonitis, bacterial infection, and blood poisoning.

A spreader was inserted and the intestines exposed, revealing a twelve-inch blockage with extensive infarction and a small rupture. This was probably caused by excessive abdominal straining, possibly due to constipation, causing a portion of the intestine to telescope into itself resulting in a blockage, reduced blood supply to the tissues and a great deal of pain. Eventually the involved section of intestine became necrotic from lack of oxygen and nutrients, the walls became friable and small tears appeared, allowing ingested feed to enter the abdominal cavity and resulting in complications and death.

Dr. Friedson and Dr. Branberg agreed that further surgery and treatment would not save the ewe and euthanasia was the humane thing to do.

"Even if we do a complete resection and successful anastamosis, I doubt if she would make it," Dr. Friedson said, taking off the rubber gloves. "She's too toxic and the infection is too extensive."

"Well, she's already terribly weak," Dr. Branberg added. "I don't think she would survive the surgery, let alone overcome the other complications."

"Let's just put her down and tell Mr. Pierson what we found and that it was our professional opinion that it was best just not to let her wake up. He wouldn't want her to suffer."

A life-ending solution was injected into the right radial vein and within seconds the respiration ceased, the heart gave up and the body lay motionless. Dr. Branberg called the Piersons and gave them the sad news.

Stew Amsey began to feel a little uneasy because what started out a couple hours earlier to be a comical situation involving him was turning into a serious and sad situation. Mr. Pierson had just lost one of his special ewes and he was bound to be confused, frustrated, and justifiably angry. He had been given false hope. He had been assured that his Bonnie would recover even before an examination was made. He had been told a sheep specialist would be tending to his ewe so she would be in excellent care. The doctors did not try to correct the problem to give the ewe a possible chance to live. The ewe was euthanized without Mr. Pierson's permission, and he had no opportunity to be with her at the end. Mr. Amsey, an innocent bystander, was at the focal point of the whole scenario.

Dr. Branberg drove out to the rundown farm and while standing in the barn watching Mr. Pierson bottle feed a newborn calf, he confessed that Stew Amsey was not a veterinarian. He tried to explain the seriousness of the sheep's condition, was sorry for his insensitivity towards the situation, and confessed his negligence for not contacting Jon before putting the ewe to sleep. He was sincerely apologetic and begged forgiveness.

Mr. Pierson showed no sign that he heard a word that was said or that he was even aware that anyone was present and conversing. He stood silently straddling the wobbly calf, holding the nipple in its mouth and softly scratching its back. When no response was given and no recognition was evident, Dr. Branberg got into his car and drove back to the hospital.

A week later Rachel walked into the laboratory and laid a short letter on the table in front of Dr. Branberg. "Maybe this will teach you a lesson," she said coolly, standing with her arms folded. He picked it up and slowly read the shaky handwriting.

"I be much disappointed and sad about the thing that happened last week about my sick ewe. You were not honest with me and lied when you said a sheep doctor would save her for me. I no longer trust you as my doc for my animals. I will call another vet to come to my place. Do not send a bill." The letter was signed Jon Pierson

THIRTY ONE

I t weighed heavily on Dr. Branberg every time a client expressed dissatisfaction with his services, and today was no exception. He had a restless night beating himself up for how badly and unprofessionally he had handled the Pierson case. As he tossed and turned, he went over the events of the day. He had lied about Stew Amsey being a sheep specialist. He was at fault for giving Mr. Pierson false hope. He was negligent in not examining the ewe before giving a prognosis report. In hindsight, he should have performed a resection and intestinal anastamosis to try to give the patient a chance to live. It was insensitive of him not to call Mr. Pierson and let him make the decision on euthanasia. Everything could have and should have been done differently and if it had, now he would probably have some peace of mind and maybe have retained a good and longstanding client.

The following morning he was still wrestling with his thoughts when he pulled into his parking spot behind the hospital. He frowned as he noticed Dr. Friedson's car sitting with the trunk lid up and both back doors wide open. It was too early for cleaning and restocking; he always did that in the evening. He sensed something unusual was happening.

"You better check with Dr. Friedson, he's been up and out early this morning and he probably needs your help," Rachel said as she met him at the door.

"Did he have an emergency?" he asked.

"Joe Baler called him about a lot of sick cows," she replied.

He walked into the pharmacy and found Dr. Friedson putting 500ml bottles in cases and stacking them against the wall.

"What's up?" Dr. Branberg asked nonchalantly.

"Joe Baler has several acute cases of what I am sure is engorgement toxemia. It appears his milk herd broke into a cornfield last night and he has Holsteins down everywhere. I would appreciate it if you would come with me. We will need a lot of glucose, all the EDTA we have and several IV sets. Perhaps you could stop by Hanson's and pick up a few sets, if they have any. We have to hurry. Some of those cows are in bad shape. Joe was going to call his sisters to come and give us a hand."

When the doctors pulled into the barnyard, the three sisters were sitting on the tailgate of an old Ford truck putting on boots, and one had put on a pair of bib overalls and had her hair tied up in a blue bandana. Joe came walking up from the milk house and leaned against the box of the truck.

As Dr. Friedson was putting on his coveralls, he looked at the small group and said, "Okay, here is the situation. We have many cows acutely sick with engorgement toxemia, meaning they are bloated and poisoned from eating too much of something rich that they are not used to: in this case, succulent green corn stalks. If they aren't properly treated, and soon, they could die and those that don't could have serious lasting effects."

He walked over to the women, and looking them squarely in the eye said, "This is the plan of action. We work on the downer cows first because they are the sickest and need immediate help. We have to pass stomach tubes through their mouths and into their stomachs to expel the gas from the rumen to reduce the pressure on the diaphram and ease the breathing. This will also slow down the rate of toxins absorbed into the blood stream. Dr. Branberg and I will pass the tube and you ladies will hold the tubes in and work them to expel the gas." Dr. Branberg came from behind the car carrying several rubber and plastic one half inch, six foot long tubes.

"After the worst of the cows are out of danger from bloat," Dr. Friedson continued, "we have to administer large amounts of glucose and a special detoxifier intravenously to all the cows. You will have to help us get props to tape the bottles to so we can monitor the flow of the liquid."

The cows were laid out all the way from the field to inside the barn. The ones that were still on their feet were staggering, walking in circles and having a hard time maintaining their balance. Most of the cows were showing various degrees of bloat and some of the downer cows were so bad their tongues and lips were turning blue.

Metal mouth speculums had to be used to pass the stomach tubes because the animals were in so much pain they were grinding their teeth and would chew the tubes in half. After the doctors passed the tubes, two of the sisters worked them back and forth to expel the gas from the rumen while Joe and his other sister were instructed to place the rubber IV sets on the bottles of glucose and tape them to anything that would support them about three feet above and near the downer cow's head. A pitchfork stuck in the ground was a good support for bottles for cows who were not near a fence. For the downer cows in the barn, they used the stanchions, posts, rafters, and milk pipes. Along the road to the field they used fence posts and the barbwire fence. In the field they used sticks, boards and metal rods.

When the worst of the bloat cases had been stabilized, the doctors began inserting a 16 gauge needle into a jugular vein of each cow and rapidly running 5% glucose into the circulatory system. This would help to dilute and neutralize the toxins and serve as a carrier for the EDTA detoxifier that was injected into the glucose through the rubber tubing. Joe's sisters monitored the infusions and notified the doctors when the bottles were empty and the sets ready to be moved to the next cow.

The next step was to get the standing and walking cows into the barn and locked into the stanchions to be evaluated and started on treatment according to their condition. Joe counted thirty Holsteins that needed to be stanchioned besides the eighteen that were down and being treated. Some of the cows went down while being herded up to the barn and had to have assistance to get back on their feet. A few were too weak to get up and keep their balance and had to be treated where they went down.

The six people worked well as a team, and Dr. Friedson was pleased with the progress being made and how well the cows seemed to be responding. He was still patting himself on the back when the oldest sister leaned through the back door of the barn and said, "Dr. Friedson, there is a cow lying on her side down by the gate. She is breathing quite heavily." After a quick look, Dr. Friedson ran to his car, found a trocar and hurried back to the cow. He palpated a spot on the left flank just posterior to the last rib where the rumen presses against the skin, and sharply stuck the trocar into the stomach. When he withdrew the probe from the metal tube, large amounts of gas escaped with a shrill whistle, spewing foul-smelling green fluid and pieces of corn and grass several feet into the air. The pressure on the cow's lungs was reduced as the gas was expelled and her respiration slowly returned to normal. Her blood was oxygenated and she would live to see another day and maybe return to the milking string.

It was estimated that 62 cows had been in the cornfield, some much longer than others. Eighteen were considered critical and treated for bloat and given large doses of treatment intravenously. Thirty were treated only for toxemia, while the remainder was put under observation. Altogether the doctors used 66-500ml bottles of 5% glucose, an undetermined amount of EDTA powder,

9-100ml bottles of penicillin/streptomycin combination and four hours of their time.

Dr. Branberg had matters to attend to at the hospital and left Dr. Friedson to complete the treatments, give a final evaluation of each cow and do the cleanup. However, the Baler family's work was just beginning. All the cows had to go into the milk barn and have their udders stripped out by hand into milk pails so as not to contaminate the milking equipment with the tainted milk. The milk would have to be discarded due to the toxins and antibiotics circulating through the blood and into the udder.

The whole incident was going to be a great financial loss to Mr. Baler, not only in the loss of milk production, but also in the cost of feed and supplements to bring the weakened cows back to good health. In a month he would get a pretty stiff bill from the Valley Veterinary Hospital.

THIRTY TWO

When Alton arrived at the clinic the next morning, he was surprised to see Dr. Branberg working in the lab.

"What are you doing here?" he asked. "I thought you would be gone by now."

"I wanted to finish these mastitis slides. Wiser's cows should be treated this week and I wanted to start another batch of acidophilus milk. We seem to be getting a lot of calf diarrhea and I don't want to run out."

"I thought your plane left this morning and you would be on your way."

"No, we leave at 2:00 p.m. Cherise will take me to the airport later this morning. The plane gets into Guadalajara around 5:30 p.m."

Dr. Branberg loved Mexico and had made friends with several veterinarians in central Mexico. He had taught himself Spanish and made a trip to Mexico once a year on the pretense it was a business trip to cement international relations through the veterinary profession. It really put the pressure on when one of the doctors was gone, but they both realized the importance of vacations and the chance to get away for some rest and diversions.

"Before you set your schedule, you should know that Matt Riddel called a few moments ago and said he has a heifer that has been trying to calf since 5:00 a.m. He may call soon. If she's a heifer and hasn't popped by now, I think you will have your hands full," Dr. Branberg said.

The phone rang as Alton was walking to the front desk to check the daily schedule and he heard Rachel say, "Okay, Mr. Riddel, I'll tell the doctor. Dr. Branberg is gone but Dr. Friedson will be on his way."

Because the hospital's horse clientele was growing rapidly, Alton found himself taking fewer dairy calls than he did when he had started in the practice. Time just didn't allow it. But when the opportunity presented itself, he was ready and willing. It gave him a chance to see friends he may not have seen for awhile and after all, it was only a few years ago that dairy had been his first love. He felt confident, experienced, usually had good results and the dairymen liked him. So he was in good spirits as he drove out to see Matt and deliver a calf for him.

Matt Riddel operated a small dairy farm all by himself. He had no hired man and worked a good fifteen hours a day. He milked fifty cows using a double string in a stanchion barn with an inline piping system. His dream was to have a milking parlor with the latest time-saving DeLaval milking equipment, but he wasn't young and probably wouldn't live long enough to enjoy it.

Matt's cows were not top producers but they were healthy, clean and happy. He kept the barn and loafing sheds clean and fed the cows high quality feed. He was a hard worker and was always around, but Alton noticed he had one peculiarity: he seldom participated in the treatments when veterinary services were required. He always had the cows and calves confined and showed the vets where they were and what ailed them, but when the work began he disappeared. Today was no exception. He barely looked up while switching a milk machine when Alton walked through the door. He was squatted between two cows when he shouted,

"She's in the calving pen. She's been straining for at least three hours. She's a young heifer."

Dr. Friedson filled his bucket with hot water, picked up a box of plastic sleeves, a bottle of lubricant and headed for the shed. As he stood looking at the heifer, he knew he had seen this scenario many times previously: the semen from a large bull artificially inseminated into a small heifer who is now trying to give birth to a large headed, heavy boned calf. The combination ruined many good heifers and yet some dairymen just couldn't put two and two together. Agricultural Extension people were encouraging them to breed their heifers to small beef bulls, like an Angus, to avoid problems, but the retort was that the calves would be worthless. So here he was, looking at another beautiful, well-bred heifer with the possibility she would never bear another live calf.

During the process of turning, twisting and pulling, trying to get a big calf out of the uterus, serious damage can be inflicted to the uterus, the cervix, the vagina and pelvic tissues to the extent that the cow may never again conceive or carry a calf to term. Sometimes the pelvic nerves are so badly damaged that the cow is permanently paralyzed. Alton hoped this was not the case this time.

He locked the heifer's head into the stanchion, tied her tail up over her back and around her neck with a piece of twine, and washed her buttocks area with Iodex. He lubricated the plastic sleeve and inserted his hand and arm into the vagina. Immediately he was confused. He felt no nose, no head, no feet, and no tail, just a mass of muscle and hair. It was as if the calf was presented sideways, but that was impossible because the uterus wasn't wide enough.

While applying more lubricant to the plastic sleeve, Alton whispered to himself what he suspected and inserted his arm again to verify his suspicions. He ran his hand along the upper portion of the uterus searching for the calf's neck, then slid it down the left side feeling for the vascular groove running along the bottom of the neck. His suspicions were confirmed. The calf's head and neck were twisted sideways and lying tight against its right side. Both front legs were folded down against the calf's belly - virtually a round ball of hair and flesh being pushed against a much smaller oval opening. With such an abnormal presentation, it would be impossible for the calf to be born without assistance and after such a long time of labor, even the best effort probably would not save its life. Dr. Friedson knew what had to be done to save the cow's life, but first he had to make another positive examination. He inserted his hand, located the carotid artery and waited for the life giving pulse. There was none. After nine months of developing, growing, and maturing, the young calf's life was snuffed out in just a few hours.

On his way back to the car to get the necessary equipment for the job at hand, Alton stopped in the barn to break the news to Mr. Riddel and ask him if he could give some assistance.

Apologetically he stated, "Well, I just started this second string so it will be about an hour. I can help you then."

Alton knew Matt's answer even before he asked the question. As he walked out the door he shouted back, "Well, I'll do what I can."

He took the fetatome out of the case and uncoiled a new cable saw from the packet. Removing a fetus piece by piece from the uterus of a cow isn't easy and to have to do it without help made it even tougher. He fastened one end of the cable saw to a metal handle, and then ran the other end through a twenty-inch piece of metal tubing to be inserted into the heifer's vagina. That was the easy part. The hard part was to manipulate both hands into the uterus and maneuver the other end of the cable around the part of the calf that was to be excised. The cable would then be passed through a second metal tube and fastened to another metal handle. The tubes would prevent the cable from cutting into the sides of the vagina during the sawing action.

By pulling and moving the cable back and forth, Dr. Friedson was able to remove the calf's head making it possible to successfully maneuver the body of the calf into the birth canal

At this point the heifer was so exhausted she didn't really know what was going on and didn't have the strength to offer much resistance. So with not much of a struggle, Dr. Friedson was able to pull the calf from the uterus much to the relief of the heifer and himself.

Dr. Friedson inserted four urea boluses into the heifer's uterus, untied her tail and released her from the stanchion. She would be swollen, stiff and sore for a few days and would hopefully expel the placenta within 48 hours. In three days or so she would come into her milk and could join the milking string and be bred again when Matt thought she was ready.

As Alton was cleaning his equipment, Matt walked into the milk house and quickly said, "Sorry I didn't make it out to help you. Did it go alright?"

"I had to cut the calf out but the heifer is okay. If she doesn't clean in two days, call me. I don't want that afterbirth in her too long. There are potential problems already without her being toxic and sick. I left her in the pen."

"Thanks," was all Matt said. He stood for a minute, then left.

"It was a bull calf!" Dr. Friedson shouted after him.

THIRTY THREE

When he got down the road a ways, Alton called into the office and smiled when he heard Rachel's pleasant voice. She always seemed less pressured and more at ease when Dr. Branberg was on vacation. Not that they didn't get along, it just seemed that she felt under the gun when he was pacing around the hospital. He was the type of person who could not quite make up his mind and it kept her hanging. She would push for a decision so she could get on with her work, but he would just mumble, pace and scratch his head. She would smile, roll her eyes and wait.

"Where have you been? It's almost noon," she asked with a little authority in her voice. She was now the boss of the office and felt she could throw her weight around.

"I'm just leaving Riddel's. I had to cut the calf out. It was a bull calf so really no loss. I'm on my way in."

"You have to swing by Price's. Melissa is taking her pig to the fair and needs a health certificate. As long as you are driving by, you may as well do it now. I told her you were out that way and she is expecting you. And Edna MacDonald called and wants you at her place at seven o'clock sharp. She has three goats to dehorn and the moon is just right tonight."

Although Edna had been a longtime client, Alton had never been to her farm. When she called she made it clear that she wanted Dr. Branberg and would wait until he was free. Today she had no choice to accept Dr. Friedson because Dr. Branberg was gone and by the time he returned the moon would be out of phase.

Edna had a few acres just east of Bear Lake. She loved her small menagerie of animals: two cows to provide for milk and cream, chickens that give her a dozen eggs a day, a few goats to chew down the weeds and blackberries, and several dogs and cats to scare away the mice and keep her company. Once a year she had to have her new young goats dehorned and have the males castrated. She firmly believed that the phase of the moon controlled the flow of blood in an animal's body. During the new moon there appears to be less blood in the animals head and more in the legs, so this was the time to dehorn. During a full moon much of the blood is in the head, neck, and chest, so that was the optimum time for castrations. Tonight must be a new moon.

Mrs. Price was not one to spend much time in the barn even though she was married to a gentleman farmer and all three of her kids were very active in FFA. She didn't like the smell of the pig pens, and she claimed if she got pig manure on her shoes she could smell it for weeks even though she practically ruined them scrubbing with every cleaner imaginable. She said the pig to be examined was in the first pen on the right, and he could stop by the house with the required health certificate.

Dr. Friedson had no trouble finding the pig in the pen but it was no ordinary pig; it was a boar. And not just any boar: a huge Hampshire boar he estimated to weigh around eight hundred pounds. He had no fear getting into the pen with the boar because being an FFA project, he would be friendly and accustomed to people handling him. Alton went through the steps of examining the ears, eyes, mouth and, of course, the snout. He was fascinated by a pig's snout. It was so versatile, useful and peculiar that he likened it to an elephant's trunk. He ran his hands along the back, down the sides and down the legs and was again amazed how stiff and prickly a pig's hair can be. He looked around the pen and kicked at a pile of fresh manure. It appeared normal, with the distinctive smell. So Alton assumed the boar had a good appetite with no sign of diarrhea or intestinal disturbance. He was about to leave when it struck him that this was a mature boar and was required to have two fully developed testicles in order to be entered in a show. He walked behind the boar, and as he reached down to pick up the scrotum, the monster stepped backward and stood right on Alton's foot. He let out a scream and gave a rough shove, but he may as well have pushed against a cement wall. The pig just grunted and stood pat. Two hundred pounds of two sharp pointy toes pressed into Alton's instep. He kept screaming, pounding on the pig's back and pushing with his whole body but the brute was stubborn. He tried to grab the top rail of the pen and pull the pig over, but he couldn't reach it. He pulled on the pig's ears and twisted its tail, but the pig seemed to like it and stood perfectly still hoping for more affection. The pain was excruciating and he was sure a few toes were already broken. As a last resort, he reached over, emptied the plastic water bucket and began beating the boar on the butt, then its back and even on its head. As before, the boar must have interpreted this also as a sign of affection. He just stood there with a pleasant look on his face.

Suddenly an idea struck Alton, and if he had had two good feet he would have kicked himself. Being a male himself, he was aware of how sensitive the testicles are. A small amount of pressure is quite painful. That is why the pig moved in the first place - he was aware that Alton was going to squeeze his prize possessions. Slowly Alton slid his hand down and with a strong grip grabbed the huge right testicle and squeezed with all his might. The boar let out a loud grunt and lunged forward, but in doing so, he put what Alton felt was eight hundred pounds on his hind feet and right on Alton's already busted foot. Alton fell against the pen, reached for the water bucket and sat down. The pig swung swiftly around and stood looking at him as if to say "How dare you!"

Alton hopped around the pig and out of the barn and delivered the certificate to the house. At the end of the driveway he stopped the car, opened the door, turned around and took off his boot. His horse doctor's opinion was that the foot wasn't broken, just badly bruised. "If I never have to wrestle another pig it is okay with me!"

Suddenly the radio clicked on. "This is 963 calling 201. Dr. Fried, where are you? You should have been in an hour ago. Are you enjoying yourself at the coffee shop or something?"

Dr. Fried didn't have the wherewithal to answer.

THIRTY FOUR

E dna MacDonald's farm looked tidy but cluttered. It appeared as if there was a fence, a shed, a small piece of machinery or animal on every square foot. When Alton drove into the yard, she was sitting on the porch with two Border Collies and didn't get up until he was out of the car. His first surprise was that the two dogs didn't run barking to the vehicle to announce his arrival. They were very well behaved.

The second surprise was Edna herself. Alton knew she was Scottish so he expected to meet someone quite husky, wearing a long skirt and barking out orders with a deep mezzo-soprano voice. Instead he introduced himself to a rather small woman with a clear, pleasant voice and wearing bib-overalls. He didn't know why, and it didn't make any difference, but he liked her immediately.

"Hello, Mrs. MacDonald. I'm Alton Friedson. We haven't met but Dr. Branberg has spoken of you," he reached out his hand and felt a little embarrassed for addressing her as Mrs., but he wasn't quite sure what salutation to use.

"Edna, call me Edna. Yes, Dr. Branberg is my preference when I call for a veterinarian. He is the only one who has been here in the past twenty years. Of course, it is only once or twice a year as my pets seem to keep themselves quite healthy and out of trouble." Pointing to the dogs she said, "These are my helpers: Salt and Pepper. I couldn't run the farm without them."

Looking around, Alton complimented her by saying, "You have a very clean, orderly place here. It looks nice."

"Thank you. It's not very big and I find if I work at it a little each day, it is easy to keep it this way."

"I suppose the young lady in your office told you what I need," she continued. "I breed Nubian goats and once a year I have to have their horns removed and the boys have to be fixed. I have four young ones this year and, unfortunately, two are males. You might think me a little off my rocker and I suppose Dr. Branberg has told you so, but I am adamant about doing these procedures when the moon is in the right phase. I have followed this rule most of my husbandry life and have had no trouble. Dr. Branberg accepts my peculiarity and has done a wonderful job over the years. I highly respect him as a veterinarian," she hesitated for a moment, "…. and as a person."

As they walked to the first wooden gate, Alton thought of the other single, elderly women who worked and managed small farms in the county. Anna Kerner came to mind; a single woman in her seventies who owned and operated a dairy farm all by herself. She milked twenty cows twice a day, cleaned the barn, washed and disinfected the equipment, delivered and cared for the calves, raised a big garden, and kept a tidy household. She even had time for baking. After the job at hand, she always invited the doctor in for coffee and a fresh pastry. Edna and Anna were very much alike.

The goats were small and the horns were just nubbins. The task would be quick and simple if Edna would agree to what Dr. Friedson was to propose. After looking at the goats and feeling the horns and the males' testicles, he squatted on his knees on the straw and looked up at her with a serious expression. "I know Dr. Branberg has been here many times and has used the same procedure to dehorn and castrate for many years with great success, but medical procedures do change, and usually for the better. I assume Dr. Branberg has removed the horns either with a gouge or a calf dehorner and has castrated the boys with a scalpel and an incision. Am I right?" He looked at her, expecting an affirmative answer.

"Yes, that is the only way I have seen it done," she replied.

"Well, those methods have been very effective and got the job done. But there usually is some bleeding, there is the possibility of infection, and the wounds are the perfect setting for flies and maggots, not to mention the lingering pain and discomfort. I was hoping you would consider a different method for both procedures."

Edna stood looking down and petting the head of the nearest goat. "By the way, this is Zane. I love the Zane Grey novels and think Mr. Grey was a talented writer. So in his honor I named this magnificent specimen Zane. She shook the goat's head and pulled his ears. "Well, I am not against progress, but I am not one to fix something if it isn't broken. New things and new ways are not always better, maybe just more convenient, faster or maybe just labor saving. I don't stand in the way of progress but I don't always agree with it or accept it."

"If you didn't go along with or accept new ideas, you would still be riding horses, using kerosene lamps and sending smoke signals," he offered with a smile.

"To be honest, those days weren't so bad. So what do you wish to propose?" She responded.

"That we use a designed hot iron and burn the horns off. It inflicts about the same amount of discomfort as the knife but there is no bleeding, no open wounds, no fear of infection, and the young animals tolerate it quite nicely. The heat cauterizes the nerves and vessels and the nubbin buttons will fall off in a week or so. And the good part is, you don't have to wait for the right time of the moon."

He gently took the little goat in his arms and rolled him over on to his back. Taking hold of the little scrotum he separated one of the cords and said, "There are small cords, tubes, and vessels that come down from inside the body into the scrotum. With an instrument called an emasculator I can quickly crush those tissues and the testicles will gradually shrivel up and die. There is very little pain, no open wounds, and no bleeding. There is nothing to see and nothing to do. Both procedures on little Zane here will take less than two minutes."

"I guess it won't hurt to try it. Zane can be the guinea pig, or guinea goat, so to speak. Do you need anything besides my help?"

"A bale of hay to stand the boys on. It's easier to work on them if they are not so close to the ground. I'll go get my things. Oh, I will need electrical power to plug in the iron."

As he walked back to the truck Alton wasn't sure he was doing the right thing. On the medical side he knew the procedures he was proposing were for the best, but how would Dr. Branberg feel about Dr. Friedson moving into his territory and making changes? The next time Dr. Branberg made a call, would Edna expect him to use the hot iron and emasculator or would she not say anything and deal with the blood, the open wounds and the worry of complications? Perhaps Alton was stepping out of bounds, but this wasn't the first time.

When he returned, Edna had plugged in an extension cord and had a bale of hay sitting squarely in the middle of the walkway. He plugged the clippers into the cord, then turned to Zane and said, "Okay, buddy, I guess you are first." He motioned for Edna to lift him onto the hay bale.

At first the clippers scared the little guy, but as Edna spoke soothingly to him he settled down and soon Dr. Friedson had the hair clipped off around the top of his head. "You look so cute," Edna purred as she kissed him on the nose.

As Dr. Friedson unplugged the clippers and plugged in the iron, he said, "Now put your arms around his neck and take a firm hold. Whisper sweetly into his ear. I'll tell you when I am going to squeeze and he will jump a little and might even bleat, so be prepared." With his left hand Alton reached down, found the scrotum and with his thumb and forefinger found the cord and vessels and pressed them against the side of the scrotum. He then carefully placed the emasculator over them and put just enough pressure on the handles to keep everything in place. "Okay, on the count of three. One, two, three!" He squeezed the handles together, felt the crunch and felt Zane tense a little. One side was done.

As he removed the instrument, Edna said, "Hurry and do it. I'm ready. I thought I heard you say three."

Alton smiled, "It's done. He took it like a trooper. But I have to do the other side."

"You mean he didn't feel it?" she asked surprised. "He didn't jump or yell. He must have felt it. He couldn't have liked it. That is simply amazing. Doesn't it hurt at least a little bit?"

"Well, he's just a little guy and the vessels are very small and soft. The pressure is on for only five seconds. Beside, he's tough. Ready for the other side? Take a hold. Here we go, one, two, three."

She wanted to see what the area looked like, so Alton stood Zane on his hind legs and she took a peek.

"All I see is a fine bruised line. I am impressed. Is that all there will be?" she asked as Dr. Friedson put the goat down.

"Tomorrow the crunch line will be black, then it will disappear, the little testes will shrivel up and be absorbed and Zane will never be a daddy."

"It certainly is different. We may as well do the others as long as you are set up. I like it, but I will hold judgment for a few days."

They did the other three goats, Curly, Zoe, and Nancy, and finished without a hitch. The only negative comment Edna made was about the unpleasant smell of the seared flesh from the hot iron on the little horns. Dr. Friedson gathered up his equipment and as he leaned over the stall for one last check, he said, "You won't have to check them through the night, they'll be alright." He had to say it even though he was sure she would be out there several times - they were her children.

Dr. Friedson thought twice before bringing up the next subject but felt it was his professional responsibility to do so. As they walked through the gate, he said, "I don't want to alarm you, Edna, but I have to say that castration by emasculation is not always one hundred percent successful. In a few instances a testicle will not shrivel up, die and go away. If this happens, there is a logical explanation. It is usually one of three things. The person doing the procedure may be incompetent and will let the artery slip out from the emasculator, and it won't get crunched and the testicle remains alive and viable. Or the emasculator may be old and warped and can't close tight enough to properly do the job. Thirdly, if the animal is big and not young, the tissues are too thick and strong to be completely severed and the procedure fails. When you read the statistics about the percent of failures, it includes all the animals done. My guess is that all the missed ones are the old bulls. At this time I am not concerned. The castrations went well and I am sure there will not be a problem. Don't dwell on it."

"And if there is a miss, what do we do? Try again?" she asked.

"We'll know in about two weeks," he answered.

"I would like to invite you in for coffee and a treat. I have some fresh zucchini bread. I think we should celebrate a job well done and the education I received."

"I really would like to, Edna. Dr. Branberg has told us about your excellent baking, but it's late, I haven't had dinner and my wife will be waiting. It's probably foolish to ask for a rain check as the opportunity may not present itself for me to return, but if so, I'll join you then." He gave her a smile as he opened the door to the truck.

Salt and Pepper followed her up the stairs to the porch and sat quietly as Dr. Friedson drove out of the yard.

THIRTY FIVE

I t was Tuesday and Dr. Friedson was going to have a busy, fun, and profitable day. He was scheduled to go to Evergreen Stables and perform the variety of procedures Steph Barnes had on her to-do list.

Many horse stables were popping up in the area to meet the needs of the rapidly growing horse population. Enterprising families and individuals were taking advantage of this growth and building breeding stables, riding stables, boarding stables and some boarding facilities with just a barn and pasture. People, especially children, who wanted to have a horse for pleasure, breeding, or just companionship, could rent a stall and board their horse. Some families had several horses in a boarding stable. There could be a variety of different contracts signed, depending on the time, stalling arrangements, and the financial situation of the family.

These stables were the perfect setup for Dr. Friedson. He could drive to the stable, park his car and attend to many horses without driving from farm to farm. Sometimes he spent most of the day at one of these stables working on a dozen or more horses. Customarily he would not charge a travel call to the stable unless there were only a few horses to care for and he felt he had to be compensated for his time.

Steph was in her office and greeted Alton with a loud hello and bright smile – she never seemed to have a bad day. When Evergreen opened she was hired as the manager and loved her job. For 24 hours a day she was surrounded by what she loved most – the feel of horse flesh and the smell of horse manure.

"We have a lot for you today, Dr. Fried," she said as she picked up a clip board and shoved it across the desk. "You can schedule it any way you wish but Gwen Chase would like you to pregnancy check her mare first thing because she is due in heat if she is empty. If the mare is barren she will have to call the breeder this morning."

Alton checked the list. A stud castration, a sore foot, a stifle problem, a lameness, check teeth on an old gelding, look at a weeping saddle sore, several tube dewormings and shots. He took a pen and put the list in order scheduling the castration first while the day was still cool and there weren't so many flies. Plus there wouldn't be many spectators. Not that they were a problem, but sometimes they made the horse nervous with their milling around and loud talking. However, if Alton had to perform a difficult surgery or make a rare diagnosis he secretly hoped there would be a crowd because they were usually impressed and it was good for his reputation and his practice.

Gwen Chase stood with one arm draped over her mare's back and Alton noticed she had her fingers crossed. He slid his lubricated sleeved arm into the mare's rectum and picked up the right ovary. No corpus luteum; not a good sign. He followed the fallopian tube down to the uterus, running his hand under the body and back to the cervix. No swelling there; no right horn pregnancy. He moved his hand under the large colon and over to the left ovary. Aha! A small mushy, mushroom-like growth on the posterior pole; a large CL which is a good sign. And yes, as he slid his hand along the underside of the uterus he felt a swelling. Being extremely gentle he ran his hand around the swelling estimating it to be the size of a small grapefruit, making the mare forty days pregnant.

This is when Alton likes to have fun with the client, especially if the client is a woman. He knows she can't wait to hear the answer. She is on pins and needles, yet he will purposely take his time. Slowly remove his arm, pull off the sleeve, all the time ignoring her curiosity and expressions.

"Is she Dr. Fried? Yes or no! Please is she?"

"Congratulations Gwen, you are going to be a grandma."

The whole barn erupts and there are hugs and back- slapping; congratulations all around for both Gwen and the mare.

Dr. Friedson turned to Steph, "Next the castration. Why is Sheila having her stud castrated?" he asked.

"He's getting difficult. In competition he won't concentrate, especially if there is a mare in the ring who is in heat. She was hoping to keep him intact and breed him but she can't have both a stud and a performer, so she said to have him cut. She didn't want to be here."

Steph led Honor out to the grassy paddock while Alton went to his car to get his bucket, soap, scalpel, emasculator and anesthetic. Castrations were quick and easy; the most troublesome part was the recovery from the anesthetic. Alton preferred a large grassy area so the horse had lots of room to regain his balance as he struggled to get to his feet while still feeling the effects of the anesthetic. Most studs want to jump to their feet too early and one or two persons are not strong enough to hold them down. There were times when a horse was seriously injured by falling backward or getting their legs tangled.

There were three incidences that usually drew a response from those watching the procedure. The large incision made through the skin on the bottom of the scrotum more times than not drew a loud gasp. The crunching sound of the emasculator cutting and crushing the tissues elicited an "ouch" or "wow" from many of the spectators, and the dripping of blood from the scrotum when the horse first stood up would make some of the onlookers think the horse was going to bleed to death. On one occasion, the owner of a horse being castrated fainted and Steph had to work to revive her while Alton completed the surgery.

Next came the dewormings and vaccinations. Some horses needed the whole package while others needed only one or two shots. The procedures went quickly because these older performance horses had been worked on so often they just took it in stride. They stood quietly while the tube passed quickly through their nostril, down the esophagus and into the stomach. They barely flinched as Alton slapped the needle into their muscular neck and pushed the plunger of the syringe. In a stable arrangement like this he could go through a small herd of cooperative horses in a few hours.

Steph followed along from stall to stall giving a hand if the owner wasn't present and kept a record of what was done to each horse. Dr. Friedson got a copy for billing purposes and the owner got a copy for their records.

The owner's complaint on the next horse was a lot of slobbering when eating her grain and dropping small wads of unchewed hay into her manger; typical symptoms of a horse needing some dental work. First the examination. While holding the halter Alton slipped his free hand into the side of the horse's mouth, took hold of the tongue forcing it back and out between the rear molars to keep the mouth open. This enabled him to slide his other hand into the space between the cheek and the molars.

"Ouch!" He jerked his hand back as he felt the sharp points on the lateral edges of the molars. "Boy she has some sharp ones. She must have considerable pain when she eats. Her cheeks are raw and there are sores along the edges of her tongue. She needs floating."

A horse's upper jaw is considerably wider than the lower jaw and because a horse smashes its food with an up and down chewing motion, unlike that of a cow that grinds its food, the outside edges of the upper molars do not get ground off. Because horse's teeth continue to grow throughout the life of the horse, these edges become long and sharp. To correct the problem a veterinarian does a procedure called floating. The sharp edges are filed smooth using a long handled rasp. Most horses fight the procedure, not because it is painful, but because of the noise in their head. The sounds of the rasping resonates through the head bones, the nasal turbinates, the sinuses and up into the brain making the procedure very uncomfortable. Alton liked to think they appreciated his efforts when they discovered the mouth sores were all healed and they could eat normally without pain.

The next procedure on the list required a surgery that Dr. Friedson considered to be one of the most spectacular that a veterinarian could perform. Correcting upward luxation of the patella.

Mrs. Luchen led Stringer, a big boned Appaloosa gelding, into the arena, pointed to his rear leg and said, "It's his right rear leg, Doc. I just noticed it about three weeks ago and it seems to be getting worse."

Alton walked around to the right side of the horse, looked at the leg and asked, "What do you notice Mrs. Luchen? What are the symptoms?"

"When I am riding him or sometimes just leading, suddenly his leg goes stiff as if he can't bend it. He drags the toe on the ground and after some shaking of the leg I hear a pop and he is okay until it happens again."

"Is it worse when he turns to the right or backs up?"

"I haven't paid any attention. It might be."

"Let me have him for a minute." Dr. Friedson took the horse by the halter, put his hand on Stringer's chest and said, "Back boy, back." Stringer took a few steps back then suddenly his head went up, he stumbled slightly and couldn't bend his right stifle joint.

"There, that's it!" Mrs. Luchen cried out, "that's what he does."

"When you explained the problem I was pretty sure what it was," Dr. Friedeson said exuding a little pride in his voice. "It's thought to be a genetic factor. The medial ligament holding the joint together and the knee cap in place is too short. When Stringer extends his leg, like when backing up, the ligament locks over the large condyle of the femur and is so tight it can't release."

"Can something be done for it?" Mrs. Luchen asked.

"O yes, I can fix that quite quickly."

By this time several people had gathered in the arena because this lameness is quite rare and Dr. Friedson predicted that no one there at the time had ever seen the procedure to correct a locked stifle. The bigger the crowd the better; he could impress more people. He went back to his car and came back with a bottle of Novocain, a scalpel, disinfectants, and a terrotomy knife; simple tools for a major surgery.

For the benefit of the crowd, but pretending he was making sure of his diagnosis, he made Stringer back up and turn around, causing the right stifle to lock up several times. He handed the lead rope to Mrs. Luchen and explained the procedure to her.

Dr. Friedson injected a local anesthetic under the skin on the inside of the stifle joint. He waited a couple of minutes then, taking the scalpel, made a 10mm incision just anterior to the medial collateral ligament. He inserted the flat knife, turned it 90 degrees and completely severed the ligament. There was a tearing sound, a short pop and Stringer's leg jerked upward.

"That should do it," Dr. Friedson said as he walked up to Stringer's head taking the rope from Mrs. Luchen. "Let me see what he does." Alton put Stringer through some vigorous paces without a hitch and no sign of the knee locking up or the horse being reluctant to straighten the leg.

"I think he will be fine Mrs. Luchen. Just take it easy with him for a few days." As he handed her the rope he heard one of the spectators give a short, soft clap of appreciation.

Steph said she had two other lamenesses; one was a right front leg and the other was a mystery. The horse was rough gaited and the owner didn't know why.

Alton loved it when he had to try to pinpoint a nonspecific lameness; one of the most challenging things in an equine practice. He welcomed the opportunity and prided himself in being able to make a positive diagnosis more often than not. The structure of a horse's leg is quite complex and during a performance, racing or jumping, the tissues can take quite a beating. The leg not only has to support hundreds of pounds of horse flesh, but also withstand the rigors of pounding, turning, twisting, and abrupt stops. There are a number of things that can go wrong involving the bones, tendons, ligaments, nerves, muscles, and the hoof itself.

The horse, a Quarter Horse, with a white blaze resembling a question mark, was obviously lame on the right front foot and it was so pronounced Alton was quite sure of the diagnosis even before feeling the leg. As usual he began his examination by feeling for heat or soreness in the hoof, up the lower leg, between the small bones of the knee then over the muscles to the shoulder.

Just as he suspected there was abnormal heat in the foot, a sign of inflammation probably due to an infection. Using the hoof tester he applied gentle pressure to the foot and the horse jumped a foot into the air.

"Whoa!" Dr. Friedson shouted.

"My Lord that must really hurt!" shouted the owner.

Dr. Friedson explained to the owner that his horse had a sole abscess caused by either a severe bruise or a puncture wound inflicted by a sharp object penetrating the sole; perhaps a nail or piece of wire. It would have to be opened, drained and have a disinfectant pack.

Dr. Friedson cut a quarter sized hole in the sole of the foot allowing the thick, yellow pus to escape, relieving the pressure and easing the pain. He washed the cavity with hydrogen peroxide, packed it with cotton soaked in 7% iodine, and wrapped the foot with cotton and Vetwrap. He gave the horse 20cc of penicillin and instructed the owner to keep the patient in the stall for three days. He would return to change the wrap and evaluate the healing process.

After receiving a thank you and a firm handshake from the owner, Alton turned to Steph and asked, "What's next?"

"Did you bring your lunch?" Steph asked. "It's past two o'clock, you must be hungry. If not I'll share a sandwich and a thermos of coffee with you. I think you need a break."

They sat in Steph's office eating a cold beef sandwich while discussing any subject involving horses. She told him the owner of the stable was considering an expansion program. They had a long waiting list of people wanting board one or two horses and the owner was receptive to the idea of adding more stalls. This was good news to Alton who assumed he would be the veterinarian to the new clients.

Diagnosing a non specific lameness was a true challenge to anyone including a veterinarian. When moving, the horse often had an obvious jerk in his gait but it wasn't always constant. It could happen during different maneuvers and many times there was no heat, pain or swelling in the leg or foot.. That was the case with Roper. A small, heavily muscled quarter horse with short legs and small feet. The owner, Joe Wainright, had purchased the horse six months earlier and had been told by the seller that Roper had never been sick, was perfectly sound and was as "healthy as a horse".

Joe walked, trotted, and loped Roper around the arena while Dr. Friedson carefully watched the horse's movements and willingness to work. A few signs indicated that the problem was not in the hind quarters but in the front legs. Alton noticed three things in Roper's behavior that indicated discomfort and maybe even outright pain. He was short-strided in front, jerked his head up when his front feet hit the ground, and he rocked back on his heels when standing still, as if to take pressure off his front feet. Three conditions came to mind but Alton needed a closer examination. If it was what he was thinking, Mr. Wainright was in for some bad news.

He motioned for Joe to stop, dismount, and hold the horse steady. Dr. Friedson knelt in front of the horse and took a close look at the hooves; just as he suspected. There were a series of rough, irregular rings extending about three centimeters down from the coronet band. He noticed the surface of the hoof to be dry and flaky; an indication of an unhealthy foot. He picked up the feet and saw that the heels were contracted, the frog was hard and shriveled, and the sole was flatter than normal. Alton rose to his feet, brushed the shavings from his pants and said, "I hate to say this Joe but your first horse purchase has not gone well. Roper has a case of bilateral chronic laminitis."

"You mean founder!" He looked surprised. "You are saying he has been foundered and that is why he is lame. But that's not treatable."

"No but it can be controlled so the horse has some use," Dr. Friedson replied.

"How can that be, he's only six years old?"

"Age is not a factor. It is most common in Quarter horses who are overweight, have small feet and engorge on a rich, high protein diet. Toxins build up in the feet interfering with circulation and damaging the sensitive lamina. Pressure builds up causing discomfort and pain."

"I have heard of people who have a foundered horse that recovered," Joe said, hoping for a positive prognosis.

"In an acute case yes, but not a long standing chronic case. I can make a horse like this comfortable but I doubt if he will ever be cured. I can give him cortisone, Butazolidin, stand him in cold water, rasp down the walls of the hooves, split the hoofs to relieve pressure, and put in heel spreaders. You can use Roper for short rides on flat trails but he is done as far as roping, pole bending, barrel racing, and competitive trail riding."

"Well then the guy screwed me. He said the horse was sound," Joe was getting a little angry.

"It depends on how you interpret the word "sound". He can say he meant he is fat and in good shape."

"I should be able to get my money back. Perhaps if you write him a letter describing what you found and that he sold me damaged goods."

"It wouldn't be worth the paper I wrote it on, Joe. He's a horse trader. He's probably been through the ropes many times. When buying a horse without a prepurchase exam performed by a competent veterinarian, I'm afraid it's the old hard-to-swallow saying: "buyer beware". Think about what you want to do and let me know."

The next hour was spent with Steph getting the client's names and addresses and writing up the bills. Handing copies to Steph he closed the metal billing box and asked to use the phone.

"Hi Rachel. I am just leaving Evergreen; we had a busy day," he said, sounding a little tired.

"All's well here. Dr. Branberg did the scheduled surgeries and took care of the walk-ins."

"What's on for tomorrow?" Alton asked.

"You have two surgeries first thing. A spay cat and Mrs. Jurgenson is bringing Tillie in to have the mammary tumor removed that you looked at last week."

"It sounds like it might be an easy day. Hey I may stop in Conway on the way in and have a cup of coffee." He cradled the receiver.

THIRTY SIX

G ar Zantin, a 79 year-old Dutchman, lived in a brick bungalow west of town and to see him you would think he was content to sit in his rocker by his window and watch the world drive by. But not Gar. He spent most of his day stroking, brushing, feeding, cleaning, oiling, driving, and feeling totally content working in and around his two beautiful ladies; Foxybelle and Foxyfur, both Standardbred mares. Both were out of an older mare named Fannyfox that Gar owned and bred. He raised them from foals born on his small farm and had them in training for the racing circuit.

He boarded and trained them at the small county- owned race track and rodeo grounds a half mile down the road from his house. Seven days a week he rose with the sun and hurried to do what he loved more than anything else in the world. He finished the chores and workouts just in time to go home for lunch and take a short nap before returning to the barns for the evening feeding, and tucking his girls in for the night.

Mr. Zantin was the only Standardbred breeder and trainer in Skagit County and there were no state or privately-owned harness racehorse tracks in the State of Washington. Consequently, Dr. Friedson was surprised to find out about Mr. Zantin's operation the first time Gar called him to the track. Gar was planning to take both mares up to Cloverdale, British Columbia, for the summer racing meet, and to cross the border into Canada the mares needed a Coggins test and an official Washington State Health Certificate. Alton was unusually busy the day of his first visit to Mr. Zantin's barn so his time there was quite short, formal and business-like. He drew the blood for the tests, did a quick physical examination, scribbled down the pertinent data and after a firm handshake and a quick nod, hurried off to his next call. However, on the next several calls to the Zantin barn the two of them became well acquainted and became good friends. Not a buddy, buddy type of friendship but one of respect and admiration.

Alton admired Gar not only for his general knowledge of horses, but also for his medical expertise and his common sense approach to problems, and the way he handled situations that would stress most people to the breaking point. He did all his own veterinary work using ointments, poultices, and liniments, many of which he formulated himself. The only time he needed a veterinarian was to administer vaccinations and tube deworming. He did his own foot trimming but had a Ferrier do the shoeing.

It wasn't until Alton's third visit, when he had some extra time, which he and Gar were able to get to know a little bit about each other. It was time for the horses' semi-annual workup and Gar had made an appointment for Friday morning. As the work was being done they kept up a steady stream of conversation.

"How did you do up at Cloverdale this summer, Gar?" asked Alton as he drew a dose of vaccine from a vial.

"It was interesting and I had a good time, but I didn't go up there expecting to win any big purses. I went just to be in the racing arena and I do have some good friends up there. I don't see them very often. It's not like I train with other stables. It is difficult being here by myself."

"But you have a lot of training and miles on these girls, they must be competitive at some level?"

"Oh, for sure. I could drop them into the lower claiming brackets but I can't risk losing them; they're my family. I finish in the money once in a while but at Cloverdale the purses are so small that what I get doesn't cover expenses."

"But you keep doing it so you must like it."

"I wouldn't miss it. I have this dream of raising a hotshot and beating the pants off those high fliers up north. These girls are pretty well bred but not real hot. Fannyfox had some Hambletonian blood on her sire's side and I bred her to a pretty good stud in Calgary to get Foxybelle. That mare has the breeding but not the proper training."

"Gosh for the amount you work them I would think they would be in top condition," Alton said as he hung the rubber tube around his neck and reached for the lubricant.

"O they are in good condition but they don't have a competitive spirit. They're lacking in heart, a will to win. A horse has to develop a will to win and fight to the last breath to do so. These girls don't have that."

"Is it bred into them?" Alton asked, "Or is it developed through training?"

"You have to make them want to win. You can do it by pitting them against other horses, let them win, and reward them for it – they learn to like it."

"I guess you can't do that when you are by yourself. So these ladies run around the track thinking they are out for just a morning exercise and probably think the same thing when they get into a race."

"You got it. Sometimes I think they try to be last because they are afraid to get into the mix." He laughed as he took the nose clamp off of Foxy's nose.

On the way back to the hospital Alton was having a fantasy moment. Could this be the way to fulfill a lifetime dream? Could this be the chance he has waited for, for almost forty years? Could Gar Zantin be the man to grant him a lifelong wish?

As long as he could remember Alton has loved horses and until he was about sixteen his vocational ambition was to have a string of Standardbred horses and make a living training, driving and racing. In his younger years he spent many days volunteering his time to the trainers at the local race track. He would go to the barns after school and offer to wash and brush the horses, fork hay, muck the stalls, oil harness and hot walk the sweaters. He loved every minute of it and thought he had the best job in the world. His dream was to straddle a sulky pretending to be driving the great Dan Patch down the back stretch of the St. Paul Fair Grounds to the cheers of thousands of fans who had come to cheer him on and see him win. Of course it never happened and he never became an owner, trainer or driver. But maybe now it could happen.

The next Sunday Alton took a leisurely drive out to the County Race Track knowing Gar would be there talking and humming to his lovely ladies. Alton had a proposal and he was hoping Gar would go along with it.

When Gar heard the car stop he stepped through the doorway and with a surprised look said, "Well, Dr. Friedson, what brings you out? Did I call? Do I have a problem? I know my memory is getting poor."

"No Gar, I have come to make you a proposal. I think I may have a way to make these lazy pets of yours into money-making race horses."

"I suppose you have concocted a magic potion that will give them a kick in the butt."

"No," Alton giggled a little. He looked Gar straight in the eye and said, "How about letting me drive one of the mares and we race against each other. You know, developing a winning attitude."

Gar didn't speak he didn't move he just stood staring at Alton with a blank look on his face.

Alton broke the silence, "You don't know this about me, but I grew up around Standardbreds. I worked with them as a child. In fact I have an uncle who has a stable of trotters down in Arizona."

Gar came back to life. "Who is your uncle?" He asked turning and putting his hand against the barn door.

"Orlin Lassen. He trains in Buckeye, Arizona, just west of Phoenix."

"Orlin Lassen is your uncle?" He straightened up and rubbed his chin.

"Yes why, do you know him?"

"I have not met him but I know of him. He had a couple of horses stolen from the barn up at Cloverdale two years ago. It was in the papers and the Racing Form ran articles and pictures about it."

"They were two young mediocre mares Orlin sent with a trainer to Cloverdale just to get them some racing experience. The trainer put them in a stall and the next morning they were missing. They never got a trace on them and they never found them."

"I remember the incident," Gar said, "The track doubled the security and some of the trainers started sleeping in their barns. I was a little nervous but didn't worry too much about it."

"I didn't know about it until my uncle called me and asked if I could be of some help. I couldn't do much but I did call a friend who has a few horses at the little track in Ladner, and he did some checking."

"Who do you know who has horses in Ladner?" Gar asked.

"Al Massman. We went to school together back on the prairies."

"Well I'll be." Gar took off his hat and rubbed his head.

"Then you two were in school together back in Manitoba. Al and I are good friends. He doesn't stable his horses at Cloverdale but trucks them from Ladner on race day. He has some good horses."

"Al gave me Vernon Ryes telephone number. He lives in Regina and is a member of the Racing Commission. I was hoping he could help locate Orlin's horses but he didn't have any luck either. I think, and I told this to Orlin, that the horses were stolen and sold to the horse meat packing plant in Lethbridge, Alberta. Some people make a living doing that."

"Is your uncle still racing?"

"No he passed away shortly after that. The doctor said he died of heat stroke. A high heat wave hit Arizona, his air conditioner went out and he died in his house. A cousin of mine from Reno went down and made financial arrangements and took care of his belongings."

"Getting back to you driving one of the mares." He smiled and kicked at the dirt. "You know, that might just work. Foxyfur is pretty easy going; she might just take to that. If we get some competition going between the two of them there just might be some excitement around here."

Alton looked up at Gar with a smile. Gar was a tall thin man, "But Gar, there could be some consequences. I could become a good driver and Foxyfur and I could pound you and that Foxybelle into the ground."

"That will never happen; just wishful thinking I'm afraid." He put his hand on Dr. Friedson's shoulder and they walked into the barn.

The best laid plans of mice and men are often foiled again and again; and so they were foiled again.

Only once did Alton swing up on to the narrow seat of the

sulky, spread his legs and hook his heels into the stirrups and enjoy an experience he had long ago convinced himself would never happen.

A few days after Alton and Gar agreed to work together, they harnessed Foxyfur, hooked her to the training cart and Alton took her for a drive. He decided to take it easy for the first time so he never experienced the thrill of the speed, the wind in his face, the rapid beat of the hoofs, and huffing and puffing of Foxyfur sucking in air. It was a slow trot around the track using the time to get acquainted. Foxyfur behaved herself and Alton was proud of his accomplishment and was satisfied that with some time and experience he would be up to the task that lay ahead.

Two days later, due to antiquated wiring, one of the barns on the grounds caught fire and was completely destroyed. Fortunately no horses were in the barn at the time. But due to the age and condition of the buildings and economic and liability reasons, the County Parks and Recreation Department decided to close the facility and Gar and the other boarders were given notice to vacate the premises.

Mr. and Mrs. Zantin decided to leave Skagit County and move to Indiana to be with friends and live in a harness racing community. During the goodbyes there were promises to keep in touch and even visit periodically and Gar assured Alton that he would give him another opportunity someday to fulfill his dream.

THIRTY SEVEN

D r. Friedson's first appointment the following morning was to dock the tails on four three-day-old Cocker Spaniel puppies, a procedure he didn't believe in as he considered it unnecessary and interfered with the symmetry and balance of the dog. It was done primarily because the general public didn't know any different. A Cocker had a short tail, period! Why it was done no one knew. The most common answer was that "my grandfather did it, my father did it, so I do it."

Tail docking, ear cropping, and dew claw removal are three cosmetic surgeries Dr. Friedson believed to be totally unnecessary and detrimental to the well-being of the dog. He emphatically discouraged the procedures knowing that his efforts were futile. The pet owners wanted it, the AVMA endorsed it, the SPCA didn't fight it, and the dog show associations demanded it. So what was a veterinarian to do?

Dr. Friedson approved of declawing a cat although also considered to be a barbaric decision. However, it is done not for cosmetic reasons but so that a destructive cat can remain in a home as a household pet and not ruin the furniture or disfigure the family members. There are many cats that would be thrown out of the house and abandoned if they could not be declawed so as not to tear up the house. Alton was in complete agreement with the procedure as long as it was done properly.

There are several ways to remove the front claws from a cat, and Dr. Friedson often emphatically stated, "There is no excuse for a licensed veterinarian not to be able to skillfully surgically declaw a cat so that there is little discomfort and a short post-surgical recovery period." But such was not always the case. Several times he had been presented with a recently declawed cat whose front feet looked as if they had been chewed on by a predator. How could a surgeon be so careless, unskillful and unknowledgeable?

When done properly, a declaw usually does not present any serious post-surgical complications. A tourniquet to control the bleeding is place snuggly around the leg just below the elbow and the complete nail is dissected from the bed at the first digital joint. A drop of surgical skin glue is put in the cavity and the opening is closed and the skin edges stuck together. A bandage is wrapped around the foot and the tourniquet is removed. The cat is sent home the next day with instructions to remove the bandages after three days. Within 8 to 9 days the incisions have healed and the cat becomes a welcome, nondestructive, household family pet.

Without this acceptable procedure, many cats can be extremely destructive with their clawing, kneading, scratching and tearing. In a matter of seconds they can completely ruin a set of shear curtains, a pair of nylons, a silk dress or expensive suit. Over a period of time they can shred the covering of a sofa with their so-called need to sharpen their claws. For a house cat, what is the need?

Ear cropping and tail docking can become a ticklish situation, especially when it comes to show dogs. For the average household pet the owners are not too particular about the length of the tail and if the ear pattern is not perfect they accept it. But for a show dog that is going to be entered into serious ring competition in first-class shows, a veterinarian better know the lengths and patterns for the different breeds.

Boxers and Schnauzers are easy breeds for ear cropping because their ear cartilage is thick, and the ears are trimmed quite short. There is very little post-surgical care necessary to make the ears stand straight and true. The most difficult breed for an ear trim is the Great Dane because the American Kennel Club requires the ears to be as long as possible with a thin tip and yet they must stand perfectly straight. A Dane's ear cartilage is extremely thin, making it necessary for them to wear props and braces for several weeks. Veterinarians will use cotton rolls, tongue depressors, Popsicle sticks, hair curlers, and even Tampax for supports in the ears to prevent the cartilage from bending and crimping. Because of the tight bandaging the skin edges often get infected from lack of air, inadequate circulation, and moisture buildup, which can prolong the healing process. Dr. Friedson thinks it is safe to say that most veterinarians would rather do any cosmetic surgery than do an ear crop on a Great Dane.

Dr. Friedson often thought a good trivia question would be "Who is the genius who thought up the idea of amputating dog's tails?" What was the primary reason? What were the criteria used to determine what breeds received the honor of the mutilation? When given some thought, there appears to be no set guidelines determining which breeds get in line for the beautification treatment and the reasons for doing so.

Consider: Indoor dogs such as Terriers, Schnauzers, and Poodles, who have beautiful short-haired tails, have theirs amputated and yet the Pekinese, Lhasa Apso, and Schuitzu, who have long hairy tails that tend to matt up, collect dirt and debris and need brushing and combing every day, get to keep their tails intact.

The watchdog breeds such as Dobermans, and Rottweiler's have their smooth haired tails removed yet the German Shepherd with its long, shaggy tail is an exception.

Long-haired hunting dogs like the Brittanys and Springer Spaniels get the surgery when they are only a few days old and yet the English Setters, Gordon Setters, and Golden Retrievers, who have extremely bushy tails, do not have to make the taildocking appointment.

It didn't make sense to Alton that an owner would partially or completely amputate the tail of a smooth haired, thin skinned Short Hair Pointer, Vizula, and Weimeraner and not do so to the burly, thick- haired tail of a Labrador or Chesapeke Retriever. Why the shaggy Old English Sheep Dog and not the equally shaggy Samoyed or Saint Bernard?

Another decision that Dr. Friedson questioned was Collies, Border Collies and Australian Shepherds who are out herding livestock all day, running through cockleburs, thorns, and briars, splashing through muddy sloughs and craggy ravines, yet aren't candidates for tail amputation. One would think they would be much better off without that debris accumulating caboose.

However, as someone once said, "If everything made sense then there would be no reason to wonder why."

Recently Dr. Friedson had read that the veterinarians, Humane Societies, and the Animal Rights people of the British Isles were starting a movement to ban these surgeries, and have the law in full effect by the mid 1980s: A step that maybe one day would be adopted universally.

THIRTY EIGHT

I t was August. The days had been warm and sunny for several weeks but now it was cooling off and clouding up so every old-timer in the valley knew it was time for the Skagit County Fair.

Without fail, it seemed destined to rain during the second week in August when the fair activities were in full swing. Each year the Fair Board threatened to move the date but all the other summer weekends were already filled with annual fairs and events and there were no open dates to be had. Some fairs ran late into September to avoid competing with other major events on the same weekend.

The County Fair with all the on-ground animals put an extra burden on the local veterinarians. The members of the Tri County Veterinary Medical Association volunteered their time to inspect, care for, and answer to emergencies while the animals were housed on the grounds. This, along with their regular calls and rounds, was a stretch for some hospitals. However, it was a fun time, and doctors Friedson and Branberg took their turns doing duty at the fair barns while attending to the clients in their practice.

During inspection day, usually Wednesday, when all the registered animals, birds, and rabbits had to be on the grounds no later than 10:00 pm, all available veterinarians were assigned an inspection station according to their practice expertise. The inspection guidelines were clearly spelled out as agreed upon by the veterinarians and the members of the Fair Board using the state health regulations pertaining to show animals. The list of conditions for possible rejection was sent to all the 4-H leaders with specific instructions not to let a member try to enter an animal harboring a health condition that was on the list. If there was a violation, the inspecting veterinarian was to clearly state and point out the problem to the owner who was expected to accept the explanation and take the animal home. This rarely happened however, because the animals and birds that were being brought in for inspection were not your every-day, run-of-the-mill farm animals. These were well cared-for, immaculately groomed 4-H projects that had practically lived in the house with their owners. Weeks before the fair these animals have been worked on and attended to several hours a day by caring hearts and loving hands.

As usual, Dr. Friedson was assigned to the west entry gate next to the horse barns. He was to inspect the incoming horses which was an easy task because the 4-H horses coming in were always healthy and in excellent condition. The kids were well taught and supervised by their excellent 4-H leaders. If there was a question or concern about a condition of a particular horse it would have been taken care of long before the Wednesday inspection.

The inspection check list for horses was quite short. Causes for rejection were snotty nose, goopy eyes, swollen mandibular lymph nodes, coughing, visible lameness, open sores, lice and warts. Of all the conditions on the list, the most controversial was lameness. If there was an obvious hitch in the horses gait during a run-out, the veterinarian had to determine if it was due to pain, an old injury, or a physical defect. Making it easy for Dr. Friedson was the fact that he knew practically every 4-H horse in the county and was familiar with their individual quirks and health problems.

Most inspecting veterinarians overlooked small nicks and scratches often caused by a rough trailer ride into town. Alton bragged about the quality and condition of the horses in the Skagit County 4-H program and often remarked that he could count on one hand the number of rejections he had witnessed over the years.

On this particular Wednesday the inspections were going smoothly, as expected, when suddenly there was a problem and the situation got a little out of hand and soon became quite nasty.

Marie Goodman had unloaded her Appaloosa mare from the trailer and was standing quietly in line waiting for Dr. Friedson to motion her forward. He nodded to her and she led her horse into the circle. While doing a quick visual inspection of the mare Alton learned through idle chatter with Marie that she was ten years old and this was her first year at the fair. She was a member of the Boots and Saddles Club run by Mrs. Fisher. She bought Picadilly with money earned from picking strawberries and raspberries and gift money from her grandparents. She was terribly excited but a little nervous. She had been preparing a whole year for this moment.

He listened to her praddle on as he ran his hands down Picadilly's soft, sleek neck - Preen Shampoo no doubt – over her withers, along her back and around her rump. Back to the head he parted the hair and checked for lice, looked in the ears, eyes and nose then stopped abruptly as he ran his fingers along the edge of the left upper lip. Were they small rough nodules? Maybe fly bites? Scratches maybe? He took a look and discovered what he feared – warts! He had to have time to think. He had Marie run Picadilly a hundred feet out and back while deciding what to do. He had two choices – disqualify the entry or let it pass.

Disqualification would have several ramifications. Marie and her family would be devastated, the Boots and Saddle Club would be targeted, and it would be a black mark on Mrs. Fisher. However if Alton kept quiet and let it pass and a fair official discovered it later, Alton would be in trouble for either a sloppy inspection or entering a horse carrying a contagious virus.

By the time a proud, smiling Marie brought Picadilly to a stop in front of Dr, Friedson, he had made up his mind – he had no choice but to kick her out. But how to do it. How do you tell a ten-year-old girl that her most prized possession is flawed? That 12 months of planning, preparing, and working is all for nothing? How do you easily and gently break a young girl's heart?

Dr. Friedson walked over to Mrs. Goodman and quietly told her what he had found, and what he must do. She practically broke the sound barrier with her eruption.

"You what? You've got to be kidding! What do you mean disqualification?"

"I'm just telling you what I found, Mrs. Goodman," Dr. Friedson said.

"I don't believe a word of it!" she continued.

Marie hurried to the scene dragging Picadilly behind her.

"What is it momma? What happened?"

"Don't believe a word of it, Marie," Mrs. Goodman yelled.

"Believe what? What did he say?" Marie asked.

Dr. Friedson stood quietly ignoring the crowd of people gathering to witness the uprising. Finally he said, "Now take it easy Mrs. Goodman. Listen to me."

"Marie don't listen to him. He says you have to take Dilly home – she has warts."

"Warts!" She choked on the word. "Where? When? Dilly doesn't have warts. I can't take her home. I won't. I won't go." She buried her face in Picadilly's mane and began sobbing loudly.

Dr. Friedson stood in front of Mrs. Goodman and spoke loudly so she could hear.

"Calm down, just calm down," he motioned with his hands. "Calm down and listen to me."

Alton continued, "I found several small warts on the mare's upper lip, let me show you." He walked over to Picadilly and put his hand on her nose. Marie jerked the horse's head around and screamed once more, "She doesn't have warts! I won't take her home!"

Alton was losing his patience. He didn't want to get angry and forceful but he had to get their attention and explain the situation. He stood tall and in a firm voice said, "Marie, and Mrs. Goodman, I have the authority to stamp a disqualification in big red letters across your entry form and send you home for trying to enter an animal with a highly contagious condition and that is exactly what I am going to do, unless you settle down and we talk this out. There may be something we can do but you have to be calm, rational, and cooperative."

Mrs. Goodman lowered her head as if to give in and Marie's sobbing slowly subsided.

"But Dr. Friedson I can't take Dilly home. I have worked so hard. All my friends are here. I would be too embarrassed. I have to stay." The tears welled up and she began to cry softly.

"I know Marie." Dr. Friedson put his arm around her and hugged her against his side. "You have worked hard. Picadilly is in perfect condition and you deserve to be here and show her in your classes. Bear with me and I think we can work it out. Here, sit down and let's talk about it." They sat on the grass and Alton let out a big sigh.

"Warts on a horse's nose is caused by a virus – a contagious virus spread on contact and can spread through a herd of young horses in a hurry. That is why the decision was made to put warts on the disqualification list. If you are honest with me I think you would agree that you would not want Picadilly stalled next to a horse with warts, knowing the condition is highly contagious."

"No I guess not," Marie answered looking down at the grass.

"You notice how people usually pet a horse's nose when they come up to her in the stall then they continue down the shed row petting all the noses hanging over the doors. The wart virus clings to that person's hand and is spread from nose to nose. That is what we are trying to prevent. So here is my proposal, and if you agree, I think I can make it so you can enter your classes and hopefully do well."

"O, do you think you can?" Marie asked jumping to her feet. "We agree, we agree, don't we momma?"

"Well let's hear what Dr. Fried has to say."

"I can cut off the warts so they won't be visible and cauterize the roots so they won't be contagious. Now we don't have much time so this is what you do. Just sit here and relax for about half an hour; time for these people to forget what they saw and heard, then you quietly load Dilly in the trailer and take her home. At seven o'clock tomorrow morning trailer her to my hospital. I will meet you there, remove the warts and sign your entry form. Then you bring her back here and put her in her stall."

"Now here is the important part. Just in case, and I mean just in case, I am unable to destroy all the wart virus, and I have no way of knowing until it is too late, I want you to keep Picadilly as isolated as possible without raising suspicion that something is wrong. Keep the Dutch door closed as much as possible and when it is open, keep Dilly tied to the back of the stall. When you have her out and about, keep her head turned away from people and don't let her nuzzle other horses. Now, do you understand what we are doing and why? And can you do it?"

"O, we will Dr. Fried. We will follow it to the letter." Maureen got to her feet and as she straightened herself she put her hand on Dr. Friedson's arm and apologetically said, "I'm sorry. I am so embarrassed. My behavior was totally unacceptable. I apologize profusely. It was an unexpected shock and I knew Marie would be devastated. I just lost my head and I thank you for keeping your cool and giving Marie a chance to be with her friends."

Alton smiled, turned to Marie and laughingly said, "I'll drop by your stall Sunday afternoon and admire all the ribbons hanging on the door."

THIRTY NINE

Queenie certainly was the "queen of the walk". She was a beautiful black and tan Collie with tipped ears, a long, smooth nose and dark black eyes. She lived with her owner, Marion Nettles, in a small house overlooking the West Bay in Anacortes. Marion was a widow and, except for Queenie, had no relatives or family in the area but did have a sister in Tigard, Oregon just south of Portland. The sister Gladys was also a dog lover and the two visited each other several times a year.

Queenie was Marion's pride and joy and constant companion. Marion combed and brushed her regularly, fed her a healthy balanced diet, walked her daily and talked to her as if she were her child. The only time they were separated was when Marion drove down to Oregon to visit Gladys. When making these trips it was hard for her to leave Queenie behind but for some unknown reason Queenie and Gladys's dog didn't get along and there were a couple of times when there were injury inflicted tussles which made the sisters agree it was best not to let the two dogs be together.

Because of this decision, Queenie was boarded at the Valley Veterinary Hospital whenever Marion made the trip south. The staff at the hospital loved it when Queenie visited because she was always friendly, clean, well behaved and an easy boarder. Marion had only two special requests; that Queenie get a half stick of Doublemint gum every afternoon at two o'clock, and that she get to watch Gunsmoke when it showed on television on Wednesday evenings. When given the gum she lay quietly chewing away and when she was done she swallowed it. George, the night man, always watched Gunsmoke and enjoyed having Queenie lie at his feet in his apartment and watch the episode with him. If Queenie heard the theme song come on and George was late in letting her out of her pen, she would let out a long sorrowful moan as if to say 'oh, poor me, what did I do'?

On one of Marion's return trips from Tigard she was all excited because Gladys had been introduced to a gentleman in Portland who could supposedly verbally communicate with dogs. A guy who could actually have a sit-down conversation with a dog. Gladys had had three one-on-one sessions with the man by herself as an introduction, and had an appointment in two weeks for a brief visit with her and her dog..

"Isn't it exciting Dr. Fried?" she was like a kid in a toy store. "If we qualify, Queenie and I could have sessions with him and I could find out all sorts of things that I have wondered about for years."

Alton and Rachel just looked at each other. Does she actually believe what she is saying?

"I could find out if she likes me, what kind of food she prefers, is she happy, and does she like the car rides? Hey I could ask him to ask her if she likes you guys; if she likes it here. Wouldn't that be great?"

"What if you find out she doesn't like us?" Rachel asked.

"Then we will find out what the problem is by asking the man, and we will fix it."

She hurried in to Queenie's room and jabbered on about this miracle and how they were going to get to know each other better and have a great time.

In the next month Marion made two trips to Portland to meet with this talented, charming Mr. Rathskeem who was supposedly God's gift to humanity because he could talk to dogs and clearly understand their responses. She came back all excited, riding high on cloud nine, giving the staff a blow by blow account on the progress that was being made.

As Marion drove away from the hospital with Queenie sitting tall and proud in the passenger seat, Rachel turned to Dr. Friedson and very sternly said, "You're going to have to tell her you know."

"What, and burst her bubble? You're not serious."

"She can't go on believing this guy is for real."

"What harm can it do? So the guy is a fraud, a scam artist. I agree it is against the law but he isn't hurting anyone."

"It's like stealing." Rachel protested, "He's taking money from unsuspecting people and giving them nothing in return."

"Whoa, just a minute!" Alton put up his hands and looked straight at Rachel, "What do you mean nothing? This the most excitement Marion has had in years. Look at her; she's beside herself. She's glowing. Actually, now that I think about it, I think this Rathskeem is doing the public a service."

"I think it is interesting that his name is Rathskeem. Get it? Skeem. That's what this whole thing is; a money bleeding skeem."

"Yes but he is going to make a lot of people happy."

Marion stopped in at the hospital on her way down to Portland for Queenie's first visit with Mr. Rathskeem. She showed a letter to Rachel and Alton that she had received from Mr. Rathskeem explaining the protocol. It began with a disclaimer. Our "talker with dogs" was leaving the back door open, establishing an escape route.

It read, "I want you to understand Mrs. Nettles, that some breeds of dogs are difficult to work with and Collies can be the most unpredictable and the most disappointing. The reason being, they are a very intelligent breed and I am sure you will agree with that. Because they are so smart they can think. Consequently they may decide not to cooperate, which is very frustrating and disappointing. On the other hand they can be most exciting and fun when they decide not only to answer the questions, but to elaborate and go on and on with a subject that interests them at the time. We must be prepared for, and accept, the results that are given.

The format will be as follows: I will meet with Queenie alone for about fifteen minutes to introduce myself, calm her down, and get a feeling for the mood she is in. I will ask her a few questions to establish a pattern and make her comfortable with me. Then the three of us will sit together. I will have a few simple questions to set the stage then you can talk to her through me. The session will last no more than thirty minutes because most dogs lose their focus quite quickly, and can't concentrate well enough to make it worthwhile.

If you feel you would like more conversation with Queenie we can set up another session at a later date. I will see you in a few days. Regards, Mr. Rathskeem."

Alton couldn't help but admire how Mr. Rathskeem had researched, planned and executed his scam. By the time he met with Marion and Queenie he would have a wealth of information – everything he needed to know to convince Mrs. Nettles he was for real and fleece her out of a lot of money.

Mr. Rathskeem had a clever way of acquiring information about his clients. When meeting with Gladys and nonchalantly asking questions about Marion and inquiring about Queenie, he was accumulating enough information to reel in his next victim. Requesting meetings with Marion on the pretext he wanted to explain the program to her, he was able to extract valuable information without her getting suspicious. The stage was set. Queenie would get a lot of petting and praising, Marion would get the uplifting and positive answers she wanted and Mr. Rathskeem would smile all the way to the bank.

It was a brilliant scheme and Mr. Rathskeem played it like a pro. He took Queenie into a small room with nothing but a chair and a floor mat. He had six questions and answers already written down and after giving Queenie a quick pat on the head he sat in the chair and read a book for fifteen minutes. When he stepped out of the room he said, "Well, I am happy to say Queenie and I got along marvelously. She is in a talkative mood and I think we are going to have a successful time together." He ushered them into the room and after the three were settled Mr. Rathskeem turned to Marion and said, "Queenie and I just sort of clicked. There were good vibes between us and we had a good conversation. She said she is happy to be here and is excited about what we are doing and is in a cooperative frame of mind. Not in those exact words mind you, but that is how I interpreted her side of the conversation."

"Now then Queenie, come here." He placed her in front of him and told her to sit. He put a hand on each side of her head, looked her square in the eyes and said, "I am going to ask you some questions that your mistress is interested in. I ask that you cooperate and give an honest and straight answer."

"What is the area like in which you live Queenie?" He sat holding her head and staring into her eyes. After a pause he said, "On a hill by some water."

Marion sat up straight, gasped, put her hand to her mouth and reached out to Queenie, "That is right. We live next to Anacortes Bay!"

"Queenie, what is your house like?" There was a pause. "She says it is yellow with some green on the front."

"That is right." Marion said shaking her head.

"What color car does your mistress drive and do you like

riding in it?" Another pause. "A blue car. Very good. You love the
car rides. You sit in the front seat with the window slightly open."
Marion kept smiling and nodding and couldn't believe this was
really happening. Now it was her turn. She could ask questions
that for years she wanted answers to.

"Do you love your mistress?" "I love her dearly."

"Are you happy with your life?" "It couldn't be better."

"Do you like going for walks?" "Actually I would like more
exercise; especially along the water."

"How about your diet?" "I love the treats and the table food.
A larger portion of gum would be nice."

"Do you like going to the veterinary hospital?" "I really like
the people there and the old man is very kind."

"Do you do anything fun when you are there?" "Yes I watch
horses and cows and there are some loud noises."

"How about one more Mrs. Nettles. I can feel she is getting
bored and disinterested."

"Okay, ask her this. If there is anything she could have or do,
what would it be?"

Mr. Rathskeem took Queenie's head gently in his hands, lifted
her face close to his and slowly asked the question. They looked
into each other's eyes for the longest time, and then Mr. Rathskeem
lowered his head. He turned to Marion who was sitting on the
edge of her chair, hands clasped in her lap,

"Yes?" Marion asked.

"What she really would like is a playmate."

Marion seemed surprised. She looked disappointed. Maybe
thinking that she was the only companion Queenie wanted and
needed. She reached over to Queenie and said, "Well, we'll see."

Marion related the whole series of events to the staff at the
Valley Veterinary Hospital saying she was extremely happy with
what she had heard and wasn't sure whether or not she would

go back. She gave no indication if she suspected the whole thing was a hoax. Although Alton had mixed feelings about it, he was happy for her.

As she walked to the door Alton shouted out, "This companion thing. Who are you going to find that's good enough to marry your daughter?"

"There isn't anyone good enough for her," she said laughingly, "but we'll keep an eye out."

FORTY

The phone jingled and on the third ring Alton picked up the receiver as he glanced at the clock whose bright green numbers told him it was 1:28 in the morning.

He mumbled a weak, "Hello".

"Doc this is Maurine. Early is having her baby and we think we need your help. Can you come?"

"Is she down and straining Maurine? Acting like she is in trouble?" Alton asked. He really didn't want to make a trip to the farm unless it was absolutely necessary. Like a case of life or death to either mare or foal.

"Not really but she has been in labor for some time and nothing is showing. She's sweating and keeps looking around at her tummy. She could be okay but I am a little worried." Alton could tell she was more worried than she let on.

"I'll be there in fifteen minutes." He hung up the phone.

As he drove to the farm Alton was thinking he was about to deliver another cheap, way-less-than-average foal that would just be another financial burden to a family struggling to buy shoes and put food on the table for four kids. How many such clients did he have? Thirty. Forty. Maybe more. The All American apple-pie-in-the-sky dream of owning a Thoroughbred mare, breeding her to a strong blue-blooded stud, raising the once-in-a-lifetime foal that makes it to the track winning lots of money, and making the family famous. What a fantasy.

How can it happen when a family with very little income, limited knowledge about Thoroughbred lines and pedigrees, buys a cheap, poorly bred, non-productive mare and breeds her to a low-grade stud? The result is going to be a foal with little chance to do anything more than become a 4-H project for some excited, wide-eyed thirteen-year-old girl who has dreamed of having her own horse since she was in the first grade. The rich and famous spend millions upon millions to produce the "wonder horse" and seldom achieve their goals.

The Daltons were just one family in a community of families who sacrificed many of life's comforts and conveniences and even necessities, spending most of their money on their horses, hoping for a miracle. Dalton's herd consisted of three broodmares and several of their offspring of various ages that hadn't been sold or given away. And now, they would be presented with another mouth to feed.

The family lived on fifteen acres of poor, hardpan soil which was hard as a rock during the hot, dry summer and a soupy mud hole during the rainy winter months. The house was a small three bedroom one story structure housing a family of six. The rickety barn should have blown down years ago and Alton shuddered to think that that was where the horses would be stalled during the next storm with heavy rains and high winds.

Earlymaiden was lying down in the stall; wide-eyed, breathing hard through flared nostrils, and sweating heavily along the neck and high in the flanks. The whole family was moving in and out of the stall offering support and wiping the mare's face with wet towels. The mare groaned, strained, and lifted her head as if to get a look at what was causing all the confusion. Immediately Dr. Friedson recognized the signs, knew that this was not going to be an easy delivery and began barking orders.

"I need two buckets of hot water, some towels and a heavy cooler. We need a halter on Early and get her to her feet. Maureen, wrap her tail with Vetwrap while I get my things."

The foal was in the breach position with the backside up and both hocks positioned below the ventral pelvic rim. On his first palpation Dr. Friedson was pleased to find the foal's bone structure to be small and fine with small, smooth hock joints indicating the foal to be small and probably a filly. He passed the findings on to the family and they were encouraged by the news.

As in all breach deliveries the trick is to get the foal pushed down and forward far enough into the uterus to be able to flex the rear legs and get them up and over the pelvic rim and into the birth canal. This is not an easy task, but once done, the foal will, with a little assistance, slide quickly and easily through the canal and out onto a clean bed of straw. This case was no exception; after much pushing, shoving, and twisting Dr. Friedson was able to get both legs up and presented and when Earlymaiden gave a grunt and a heave, Dr. Friedson had to catch the foal to prevent it from falling hard to the barn floor. It was a dark bay filly with two front stockings and a narrow blaze. As she lay gasping for the life sustaining oxygen she was surrounded by four curious faces smiling down at the miracle of birth.

The rest was routine. The uterus was checked for a possible twin, the placenta was examined for rips and tears or missing pieces that could be retained in the uterus and cause problems. The mare's buttocks were cleaned and disinfected and the udder was washed and massaged to stimulate milk flow. When completed, Alton knelt by the new foal and upon lifting the upper rear leg announced, it's a filly.

"I knew it!" shouted the youngest daughter, "and mother said I could name it if it was a girl. I already have a name picked out." She bent over the filly and while stroking her head she announced, "I name you Early Morning Lily."

"That's a lovely name Marta, and very appropriate I must say as it is very early in the morning." Maureen said affectionately as she put her arm around her daughter's shoulders.

Dr. Friedson gave the filly a thorough examination, soaked the umbilical stub in strong iodine, and declared her to be normal and healthy and a fine addition to the Dalton's string of Thoroughbred horses.

It was a time for celebration and everyone took a turn at oohing and aahing while complimenting Earlymaiden on her stellar performance, giving them a new filly - Early Morning Lily. It was a happy time, but somehow Alton felt a sense of resentment and sadness from the older daughter Brianna. She was not overtaken by the newborn as the others as she stood with her arms folded slightly nodding her approval.

Brianna was a beautiful young lady, blossoming into womanhood and being deprived of many of the things a girl her age wanted and needed. Alton had never seen her in anything but well-worn jeans, a variety of T-shirts and run-down shoes. Did she even own a nice dress and a decent pair of leather shoes? Alton could imagine what was going through her mind.

'Just what we need, another low-grade horse to take up residence in a pasture already overcrowded with other low-grade horses with no place to go and with no promising future. With each new addition it's the same old story. There goes the new shoes for the kids – we have to pay the vet bill. There will be no vacation this year – we need another ton of grain. The girls will have to make do with what they have – we need the Ferrier out to trim fourteen pairs of feet. Dad will have to keep the dilapidated Ford running for one more year – we need another semi load of eastern Washington alfalfa. When will it end? When will my folks realize that it just isn't working? Where is the fun, the excitement, adventure and popularity of being a young, healthy, energetic teenager?'

Every day she had to hurry home after school to help with the barn chores, give a hand in the kitchen, tidy her room, and get her homework done before going to bed. While she was stuck in this boring, tedious routine, her close circle of friends were meeting after school, laughing, sharing secrets and desires and getting involved in fun and social activities.

Alton could sense her growing resentment and disgust and as their eyes met he could almost hear her say, "Thanks for nothing."

As Alton drove along the driveway and out onto Highway 9 with the rays of the early morning sun peeking over the ridges of the Cascades, he felt more depressed than the urge to pop a cork and make a toast to a new life. The scenario doesn't change. Tomorrow he could be out to one of a dozen or more other farms delivering a new foal into a barn already overcrowded and underfed. Under-achieving thoroughbreds dipping into the family's income which could be used for more urgent needs.

But what about the dream – ah yes, what about "the dream"? America was built on hopes and dreams. The sources of energy that keep a person chugging and churning with the chance of someday grabbing the "golden ring", snaring the "golden goose", or dipping into the pot at the end of the rainbow.

Many horse-poor breeders hang on to the legend of the likes of Seabiscuit and Man o'War who were born of non-descript bloodlines, purchased for a few thousand dollars and went on to fame and fortune - something that happens maybe twice in a century. With this to hang on to, they plug away thinking this could be their place, this could be their time.

FORTY ONE

"Well, what do we have here?" Rachel asked herself as she stared into the cardboard box sitting on the step next to the back door. She turned the key in the lock and kicked the door open as she picked up the box. She set it on her desk and continued to study its contents as she took off her sweater and laid it over the chair.

She mouthed the words 'a box half full of hair - dog hair'. But, why? It's matted and dirty and smells to high heaven. Did someone clip their dog and give us the hair as a practical joke? She shook the box and poked at the bundle with a pencil and decided it was some kind of prank having to do with Dr. Fried. Probably he and a client had some kind of bet on. Because it smelled so terrible, she carried the box outside and set it on the grass by the dog run.

It was late morning and Dr. Branberg was clipping the hair mats of an ornery Peke when Rachel remembered the box and the smelly hair. "Hey Dr. Branberg, are you expecting a special package like maybe some dog hair delivered in a cardboard box?"

"Not today. I don't need any more dog hair. I have all I need right here."

"Someone left the hair clippings from a dog on our back step this morning."

"Maybe they want it checked for fleas and lice. Was there a note with it?"

"I didn't look at it real close. It stunk so badly I stuck it outside. I guess we will get some answers when Dr. Fried gets in."

"Hello 963 this is 201. Do you read me?"

"Go ahead," Rachel replied, "are you on your way in?"

"I just left Hennyson's and will be there in fifteen minutes. Do you have anyone waiting?"

"Not a client but your box of hair is here. It was at the door when I opened this morning. You're going to love it."

"I don't remember ordering a box of beer. Why would I do that? I pick it up at the corner store."

"Hair!" Rachel shouted back. "A box of dog hair. You must have made a bet or did a deal with someone. Anyway, it's here."

"I haven't the least idea what you're talking about. See ya."

"The mysterious box is out by the dog run," Rachel called out as he walked into the laboratory and set a metal box of milk tubes on the counter by the sink. He would streak and stain them later but now he was curious about the box of hair. "You'll understand why it's out there when you get a whiff of it," Rachel held her nose.

Alton retrieved the box, took it into the prep room and set it on the table. Dr. Branberg took a peek and shook his head. It was an old Kraft Cheese box about ten inches wide and sixteen inches long. Inside was what appeared to be two big handfuls of black and brown hair. Not fluffed up like it had just been cut, but like it was all stuck together. It reeked of urine and feces.

"I don't know why it's here or what we are supposed to do with it but I guess we better take a look." In saying this he reached for a long pair of carmault forceps to reach in the box to get a sample of hair.

"Are you trying to convince us that you know nothing about this whole thing or prank or whatever it is supposed to be?" Rachel asked.

"I know nothing. Honest. I'm as confused as you are. Dr. B here is awfully quiet. I would suspect he is in on it somehow. He likes a joke or two."

Dr. Branberg didn't even look up. "My hands are clean. You two will have to figure this one out by yourselves."

Alton reached into the box and as he gave a slight tug on a tuft of hair Rachel threw her hands to her face, and jumping back yelled, "O my God, get it out of here! There's something in there." She was visibly shaken.

"Where?" Alton asked.

"Down in that corner. I saw something move. Like a twitch. I swear. O my God I'm scared."

Alton reached down into the corner and with the forceps lifted a small tuft of hair. To his surprise he saw a small eye ball peeking up at him. He slowly and gently touched the eye with the forceps and it blinked. "You're right Rachel, this is a live animal."

Dr. Branberg couldn't believe it. He walked over to the box and laying his hand firmly on the hair said, "Yeah there is something there alright."

"Rachel would you please get me those heavy leather gloves from the exam room then run the sink about half full of warm water. I think I know what we have here and it is going to take some special care." He lifted the mass from the box and was surprised at how light it was. He laid it carefully on a towel and took off the gloves. He looked to the area where he had seen the eye and slipping his hand under the towel he slowly lifted what he thought to be a head. At the same time a small blob of hair raised itself up and turned slightly to the right.

"It's alive!" Rachel blurted out. "What is it Alton?" Her remark surprised everyone including herself. She never called Dr. Friedson by his first name but she was so confused, amazed, and overwhelmed she about lost control.

"I think it is a little dog. And yes, it is alive. This appears to be the head," he said cupping a round piece of fur in his hand. "It can't be very big. We have to be careful not to traumatize it. It is very cold. Is the warm water ready Rachel?"

"Yes. Should I put a towel in the bottom of the sink for it to lie on?"

"Yeah, that'll work. I am going to lower her into the water and I will hold the head while you try to loosen the hair and remove some of the matts and massage the skin. We'll let her warm up then we'll get her out and see what she is all about."

"You say she. How do you know it's a girl?"

"By the looks of things this little critter has gone through hell and is still fighting; determined to live. Do you think the pussyfooting male of the species could endure such pain and neglect? No way! Males are too weak and wimpy. It takes the toughness, the endurance, the heart and courage of the female to push on to survive and perpetuate the species; it's a female."

After an hour of warming, washing, and massaging Rachel placed, what she assumed to be a small dog, on a heating pad on the table. She proceeded to comb and blow dry the hair while Dr. Friedson prepared a bottle of warm fluids.

After a complete examination they found that the ball of fur was indeed a small dog. Alton put his hands around the small head, brushed back the hair with his left hand and saw two partially opened eyes and a small black nose. He felt the ears and slid his hand down the neck to the chest. The hair was thick and actually quite soft. The dog winced and resisted as Alton tried to stretch out the front legs but they were too weak and Alton was able to move them only about half-way. The ribs stuck out like a wash board and the spine felt like barb wire.

The rear legs could not be separated because of the matts and knots in the hair. The tail was clamped down and the longhairs were wound around the rear legs. Needless to say, the poor little thing had been sadly neglected for months. After a short discussion it was decided the dog was a Lhasa Apso mix and according to the teeth Alton estimated it to be three years old.

The plan of action was to first build up its strength with fluids, soft dog food, vitamins and healthy snacks. In a couple of days they would cut off all the hair, treat for any lice and fleas and tend to any existing sores. After that they would start a physical therapy program.

Rachel named the orphan "Hairball" and took it under her wing as if it were her child. She couldn't help but grin when they cut off all the hair and discovered the little one actually was a female. Alton puffed out his chest.

When working with Hairball there was a lot of discussion about where she could have come from, why she was so neglected, why she was brought to the hospital, and what they were supposed to do with her. Rachel had given it a lot of thought and offered her own scenario.

Hairball lived with an older gentleman who lived alone in a small house probably out in the country. There was a possibility that he was disabled, sick or just couldn't do much. He may have had friends or relatives that looked in on him once in awhile and they may not have known that he had a dog. Rachel speculated that Hairball lived in a small box or cage and the elderly man gave her food and water now and then when he thought about it, and never let her out to move about or exercise. This was obvious because her legs were stiff and her toe nails were long and curled under against her foot pads. When put on the floor she couldn't or wouldn't walk.

Rachel's guess was that a visiting neighbor asked about the dog and when he saw its living arrangements and poor health, suggested to the older man that something be done. He may have volunteered to take the dog to the hospital. Rachel had a gut feeling that sometime within the next week an anonymous person would be calling to ask about the dog.

Hairball's physical condition, attitude, and temperament improved every day. After being clipped and bathed, having her nails trimmed, a flea treatment, and some nourishing food in her tummy, she definitely felt better and made an effort to sit up and even tried to walk. Her eyes were cloudy from all the hair and goop that had collected around them, but the damage wasn't permanent and she wouldn't be blind. She was beginning to look, feel, and act like a dog instead of what at first was thought to be a dirty, smelly glob of hair.

It was a week to the day since Hairball first appeared in a box on the hospital's rear doorstep. She was feeling good and had the run of the hospital and was by now the "queen of the castle". Rachel let her out of her cage in the morning and she did pretty much what she pleased – ate, slept, begged for treats, was picked up and cuddled as much as she wanted.

She was sitting on Rachel's lap chewing on a doggie bone and was startled when the phone rang next to her ear.

"Hello, Valley Veterinary Hospital," Rachel answered.

"This is an anonymous call. I am not going to tell you who I am so you have the right not to answer my questions if you choose to do so."

She didn't recognize the voice, "I'm listening."

"I'm inquiring about the contents of a box that was left on your back doorstep a week ago."

"And how do you know about that?" Rachel asked.

There was a long pause, some sniffling some grunts, and then the man said, "I am the one that dropped it off. I was doing a favor for a friend."

"What was in the box?"

"I hope you were able to take care of it; it was a dog. It needed a lot of attention."

"I will tell you this. Yes we found the box and yes, we are taking care of the dog. She is doing very well. But why don't you tell me more about the circumstances." Rachel didn't want to give out too much information in case the man hung up. "We need some information in order to treat the dog properly."

When the man started talking, Hairball lifted her head, cocked an ear and acted as if she was listening; as if she recognized the voice. She certainly was being attentive.

"I am a neighbor and a friend to the older gentleman who owns the dog. He lives by himself and has a hard time getting around. He likes the dog but often forgets he has her. I think his memory is about gone. I think the dog went many days without food and water and certainly didn't get much care."

Rachel interrupted, "Tell me more about the dog."

"She's a little girl. A three-year-old Shitzsu named Chin. She was given to my friend about a year ago by a relative who thought she would be good for him. It was a kind thought but he is unable to take care of her."

"How are you involved in this?" Rachel asked.

"I'm Joe's neighbor." There was a pause. "That's what I call him." Rachel wasn't convinced it was a mistake. "I call on him periodically and last week when I stopped in he told me Chin was dead and asked if I would take care of the body. As I was carrying her out of the house I was holding the box next to my head and I was sure I could hear her breathing."

"Did you think she was alive?" Rachel was curious.

"I heard uneven breathing like she was working to get air, but having a hard time. I didn't know what to do so I took her to my place and kept her warm until six o'clock in the morning then drove her to your hospital, hoping you folks would do the best for her."

"And you are not going to tell me who you are or who the owner is?"

"Not now. I am calling to find out Chin's status and what has been done for her. Did she die? Was she dead? Is she okay?"

"Yes, she is alive and this is the situation as of today." Rachel went on to explain what they had done for Chin, the progress that been made and what was to be expected. She doubted if Dr. Friedson would allow Chin to go back to the original owner considering the circumstances.

"I doubt if Mr. ….uh, the owner can or is willing to care for her. At this time I question if I should tell him or just let him think she is gone and is at peace."

"My suggestion is not to say anything yet, because although Chin is doing well, she is not completely out of the woods. I think you should wait until she has a complete recovery and you have given some thought as to what her future should be."

"I agree with you, I think that is a good plan," he said.

"Just out of curiosity, how should we expect to get paid? The bill is getting quite high and we will need payment from someone," Rachel was hoping to get a name or phone number.

"Just what do you think the total will be?" he asked

"I'm not sure but it could be up to $70.00. Dr. Friedson will have to do the figures."

"Don't worry, it will be settled. Thanks again." The line went dead.

It was seven thirty the next morning. Rachel parked behind the hospital, got out of her car and as she walked to the door she noticed a bag hanging from the door knob. It was a small, brown, Safeway shopping bag tied with string and wrapped around the knob. She took it inside and opened it to find a leather collar decorated with white and blue glass beads, a silver lead chain, a light blue flannel blanket, two rubber squeaky toys and a thick envelope addressed to "The Good People of the Vet Hospital". She opened the envelope and stuck between many one dollar bills was a short letter written in a very shaky, scrawny handwriting.

It read, "Thank you for being so kind to dear little Chin. She needed help and you fixed her up. I hope she is well and healthy and having fun. I ask that you find her a good home so she can have the happy life that she has missed out on. This money may not completely cover the bill but it is all I can find at this time. God will bless you."

Rachel had tears in her eyes as she counted out the $83.00 and laid it on the counter. She stood for a moment thinking that in spite of all the ugliness and hatred in the world there was still a tremendous amount of good circulating among those who were willing to give and receive it.

She picked up the Safeway bag and briskly walked out to her car and laid it on the front seat. Then, on second thought, she put it on the floor leaving room on the seat for a soft pillow big enough for a small dog.

About the Author

Dr. Fredrickson was raised the son of a Lutheran minister in the small town of Deloraine on the southern plains of Manitoba. He received his Doctorate in Veterinary Medicine at the University of Minnesota in 1963 and upon graduation, he and his family moved to Mount Vernon, Washington, where he and Barbara continue to live and work.

Dr. Fredrickson accepted the position of associate veterinarian in a well-established mixed animal practice and provided veterinary service to a variety of family pets and domestic animals. After seven years he realized his interests were with horses, not with cows, and he opened his own veterinary clinic, limiting the practice to horses and small animals. Fourteen years later he sold the equine practice and opened the first of five small animal surgery clinics.

Upon retirement he plans to pursue a few hobbies, engage in recreational activities, and do some traveling to visit family and friends and enjoy the sights and cultures of our own great land and some foreign countries.

Dr. Fredrickson says, "Veterinary Medicine has been good to me and my family and, even after an extremely difficult day, I have never regretted my decision to become a veterinarian. By having provided medical care to many animals over the years I feel fulfilled, satisfied and content that I lived up to the statements in the Veterinary Oath. I am convinced that my time and efforts served a purpose. I am richly blessed."